A New You in 30 Days

A NEW YOU

IN 30 DAYS

Improve your looks from top to toe
in one month!

Sally Ann Voak

Michael O'Mara Books Limited

First published in Great Britain in 1994
by Michael O'Mara Books Limited,
9 Lion Yard, Tremadoc Road, London SW4 7NQ

A CIP catalogue record for this book is available from the
British Library.

ISBN 1-85479-189-3

Designed by Mick Keates
Edited by Georgina Evans

Typeset by Florencetype Ltd, Kewstoke, Avon
Printed and bound by Cox & Wyman, Reading

CONTENTS

ACKNOWLEDGMENTS

My grateful thanks to all the volunteers who helped me test the New You programme, and to my assistant Jan Long who weighed and measured them so carefully.

Thanks too, to home economist Glynis McGuinness for checking my recipes and to the three stars who helped produce the superb 'before' and 'after' pictures: make-up artist Jan Wright, hairdresser Joshua Galvin and photographer Steve Lewis.

CHAPTER ONE

YOU CAN DO IT!

I wonder if you have ever looked in the mirror and thought, 'I wish I looked slimmer, fitter ... more fashionable.'? Who hasn't! The trouble is that most of us have not got the time or the spare cash to lavish on expensive health clubs and beauty treatments. I have some good news for you: for the next 30 days, this book will become your very own 'expert', taking the place of all those clubs and treatments. I promise you that, if you follow my instructions correctly, you will become confident, more attractive, and have a much more positive attitude to life. Inside that wobbly exterior is a star just waiting to emerge. Honestly!

I'll show you *exactly* how to transform your looks from top to toe in just one calendar month. The process won't be painful, quite the reverse: you'll enjoy a simple-to-follow programme including diet, exercise, beauty and fashion tips, and psychological 'exercises' to switch you on to positive thinking.

The 30-day plan is based on knowledge gleaned from my 25 years of experience in the fashion, beauty and slimming business, as Fashion Editor of *Harpers & Queen* magazine, as Beauty Editor of *SHE* magazine and, currently, as Slimming Editor of Britain's biggest-selling newspaper, *The Sun*. Over the years I have learned that good looks are more about know-how than luck. You can be born beautiful and look a mess ... you can be born averagely attractive and look stunning. All you need is the right information and a few guidelines – and this book contains just that!

I have never believed in writing purely about theories; every one of my books is about *facts*. That's why my programme has been fully tested on a group of 15 volunteers. I advertised for them in a local paper and selected a cross-section representing women of different ages, lifestyles, and figure types. The result has been that, without exception, they have *all* shaped up, slimmed down and improved their image. You can see how well it worked for them by checking the 'before' and 'after' pictures in the centre of the book and by reading extracts from the diaries they each kept during the 30-day trial. Unfortunately, we only have room for five 'success stories', but I can assure you that everyone who took part was absolutely delighted.

Here are some comments from my super bunch of guinea-pigs:

'I feel absolutely wonderful,' says Toni Tree, our cover girl. Toni, from South Croydon, Surrey, weighed 11st 11lb when she started the programme. At 32, with two small children, she felt that she needed a whole new outlook. 'I can't praise the programme highly enough. I ate more than I've ever eaten, the exercises were fun, and the beauty treatments transformed me. I lost 16½lb in the 30 days, and had the courage to have my hair cut. My general well-being improved dramatically. Most important, it lasted. Since the end of the 30-day period, I have lost a further half stone ... and still feel great.'

Another tester, Carol Barlow, also from South Croydon, says, 'Since having my three children, I felt

I had let myself go. The programme was just what I needed to boost my morale . . . My three children joined in the exercises with me, and the perfumed baths felt positively sinful. It didn't cost me a thing, and I feel tons better for it. I lost an amazing 7 inches off my hips, which was an unexpected bonus.'

Linda Henson, who is featured on the back cover, is thrilled with her new look, 'I can now walk for miles without huffing and puffing, and I have lost inches everywhere,' she says. 'I was never very overweight, but my eating habits were erratic. Now I'm in control, and I take pride in my appearance. I've always been told I look young for my age (35), but now I feel like a teenager again.'

They did it – you can too. All you need to do is set aside 30 days when you know you can concentrate on the programme. No, you do not have to take a holiday from work or give up your social life. The programme fits in easily with work (the lunchtime recipes can be packed up and taken with you, and the exercises can be fitted in during the morning *or* evening), and the supper menus are good enough to serve up to guests.

One of my guinea-pigs, Sue Tucker from Warlingham, Surrey says, 'I had several dinner parties during my 30-day stint on the programme. The guests were very impressed with the dishes, and didn't realize they were all part of my healthy eating plan.'

However, it is probably best if you do not time your 30-day 'make-over' to coincide with a holiday abroad or a series of weekend trips. For with the best will in the world it is often difficult to expect others to cater to your food needs, and too many distractions could put you off doing your exercises regularly.

One of the best possible times to start is when you are

broke! The programme does not put any extra strain on your pocket – quite the reverse. You will feel good about yourself if you concentrate on a 'new you' when cash is short. The programme really is a marvellous morale-booster.

Before you start, you need to assess your problems with the simple tests below.

ASSESS YOURSELF

Strip naked in front of a long mirror and check out the following important points:

1. *Posture Check* Stand, sideways on to the mirror, feet slightly apart and relax. Are your shoulders rounded? Does your tummy protrude in front? Does your bottom stick out behind? Are there rolls of fat around your middle?

Now, relax your shoulders, exhale and pull in your tummy muscles. At the same time, clench your buttock muscles and rock your pelvis forward just a little. Glance in the mirror again. See how much slimmer you look!

During the next 30 days, you'll be learning just how to keep your posture in check *all* the time.

2. *Cellulite Check* Look at yourself in the mirror once more (I know this is painful, but believe me, it's necessary!). Are there lumps and bumps of wobbly flesh on your thighs, bottom and tummy? Look closer. Does the flesh look pitted, almost like orange peel? Now press it. Does the pressure of your finger leave a white mark? This is a classic indication of cellulite. Although many doctors are still sceptical about this condition, it is known that this particular kind of fat *does* respond well to a diet that is rich in raw foods plus specific massage

4

treatments. Several of our volunteers were cellulite sufferers, and they all noticed a dramatic improvement in the condition.

3. *Tummy Check* Stand side-ways on to the mirror and concentrate once again on your tummy. Does it stick out even when you are holding it in? Jump up and down. Does it wobble alarmingly? Now lie down on the floor, knees bent, feet together, hands by your sides. Push the hollow of your back into the floor, exhale and pull in your tummy. Does it look better? It should! I'll be showing you how to 'find' those long-lost tummy muscles and use them properly. This, in turn, will help ease the strain on your back and the upper part of your body, and improve digestion, bowel function and generally well-being.

4. *Bottom Check* Stand in front of a long mirror and use a small hand-mirror to have a good look at your bottom. Is it low-slung? Is the skin greyish and dull looking? Are there spots all over it? Are there two 'love handles' sticking out each side? Are your buttocks flabby? If you sit for long periods, you could have all these problems. Don't worry, your bottom will respond well to the specific exercises in Chapter Two, and to the walking programme.

5. *Bust Check* Now look at your chest. Is it droopy? Is the skin dry-looking? Are there red marks where your bra-straps cut into you? Although it isn't possible to exercise the breast area itself, it is possible to strengthen the pectoral muscles which suppport your breasts. You'll be helping your bust to shape up in the bath, and special underwear tips will also help improve the look of this area.

6. *Foot Check* Now for possibly the most neglected part of your whole body – your feet. Place each foot on a chair and look at it carefully. Is the skin dry? Are the nails ragged or ingrowing? Do your toes look painfully cramped where they have been crammed into ill-fitting shoes or wedged forward into the toe section of high-heeled pumps? Is there lots of hard skin on the back of each foot? Have the arches dropped? Can you see small corns on the little toes and soft corns between the toes? If your feet hurt, it shows ... on your face! So, part of our beauty programme will be a total luxury treatment for your feet.

7. *Skin texture Check* Put your clothes on again, or snuggle into a warm dressing gown. Now remove all your make-up. Stand or sit in front of a magnifying or shaving mirror and check out the following points. Are there open pores around your nose and on your chin, with perhaps a few spots or bumps? Are there dry patches around your eyes? Do you have fine lines (or even deep ones!) on your forehead, around your eyes, and on your neck? Is the skin on your neck crêpey?

You will find that the special beauty masks recommended in the programme will help deal with all these problems, and the diet plan you will follow will also help flush out impurities. As you progress through the 30 days, repeat the checks above and watch for steady improvement. It will happen!

8. *Hair Check* Hold your hair up to a magnifying mirror. Are the ends badly split? Does the colour seem to fade along the hair shaft, looking richer at the root, lighter at the ends? Are there signs of damage along the hair shaft itself? Now sit back and assess the overall style. Is the length truly flattering? Is there enough volume to 'lift'

your face, helping to eradicate that tired, washed-out look? Or does the style drag your face downwards? Is there a glossy sheen on your hair or does it look dull and lifeless?

You will find that your hair does improve over the next four weeks. During Week Three, Joshua Galvin, who created the Healthy Hair Programme products for Superdrug, will give tips and hints on how to change your style subtly, for maximum flattery.

9. *Weight Check* Off with that robe again, and onto the scales. Make a note of your weight, and the time of day.

During the programme, you will weigh in twice a week. This is enough to help you judge how the eating and exercise plans are working for you. Do not weigh yourself more frequently. Fluid changes in the body can give a temporarily misleading result, which can be discouraging. The weight you lose during the next 30 days will depend on your starting weight, job, lifestyle and personal metabolic rate (and this varies from person to person). We found that our volunteers who had most to lose, lost most weight. Those who simply wanted to tone up and shed a few extra pounds, did just that. The average weight-loss was 10 pounds.

For your own benefit, do not cheat when you weigh-in. It doesn't help to wobble about on one leg, move the scales around the house or wear heavy jeans one day and strip naked the next. The only person you are cheating is yourself. This could also be the moment to borrow, or invest in, some decent, accurate scales.

10. *Measurement Check* During the programme, you will measure yourself twice weekly, at the same time as you weigh in. If you can get someone else to measure

you, fine. However, it should be the same person each time. Here's how to do it yourself:

Strip to bra and pants.

Bust Make sure the tape-measure is well up at the back, and take it over your bust or chest, skimming the nipples. Bring the tape-measure around to the side, so you take the reading there, rather than in front (you could lose some 'slack' down your cleavage).

Waist Place the tape-measure around the narrowest part of your waistline. Take the reading without pulling it tightly.

Hips This is the tricky one because it is very easy to take the measurement in different places at different times and so get an inconsistent reading. Select the *widest* part of your body, around your bottom. Now measure down from your tummy button to that point. Make a note of this measurement so you can pinpoint the same spot next time. Next place the tape-measure around your hips and take the reading without pulling too tightly. This is vital if you have cellulite. You will only be able to tell if you are losing those wobbles, if you measure them properly in the first place, so no cheating.

11. *Fashion check* Finally, have a good rummage through your wardrobe. Are your clothes carefully chosen to flatter your good points? Or is the cupboard full of costly mistakes; items bought when they were fashionable but which no longer do a thing for you? Are the colours bright and cheerful, or are most of your clothes black? Do your accessories go with each outfit, or is there just a jumble of shoes and handbags at the bottom of the wardrobe which don't go with anything?

No, you will not be advised to throw out everything and

start afresh. That's costly and counter-productive. Instead, some severe pruning will take place in Week Three of your programme, and advice will be given on basic items which could help 'pull together' existing items and turn a wardrobe from 'hell' into a heavenly selection of outfits that will see you through any occasion.

NOW DECIDE WHAT YOU WANT TO ACHIEVE

The checks above will help you work out what is wrong with your body. Cheer-up. No one is perfect. During the next month, you will be well on the way to becoming the very best 'you' that you possibly can.

While working through the various checks, you have probably noticed that various parts of you are weaker than others. Maybe your hair, skin or tummy need more attention than they are currently getting. Now is the time to restore the balance. You can do it.

HOW THE PROGRAMME WORKS

The New You Programme is divided into three main parts – Diet and Exercise, Beauty (which includes skin and hair care, manicure, pedicure and massage), and Self-Image (which includes positive-thinking exercises, mood control and fashion awareness).

The programme is spelt out fully in Chapter Five, and all the recipes are given in Chapter Eight.

But before you start, you must read the next three chapters of this book which will explain the concept of the programme, and help you to become familiar with the various routines before you try to follow them.

I also recommend that you keep a diary throughout the 30 days so you can check your own progress. As you will see in Chapter Six, our volunteers did just that, and were very surprised by their own candid observations!

CHAPTER TWO

A NEW APPROACH TO DIET AND EXERCISE

This is not a book about crash dieting or vigorous exercising. The New You programme does not aim to help you shed the maximum number of pounds and inches in the shortest possible time.

I believe that it is dangerous and counter-productive to force your body to follow a regime which is so rigorous that it punishes rather than educates. Instead, I will introduce you to an exciting, imaginative fitness and eating routine which you can stick to for the rest of your life. Yes, you will certainly lose weight and shape up but (sorry!) there is no chance of shedding 25 pounds or dropping four dress sizes in the four weeks. Results will be personal and they will be fairly spectacular, but there will be no miracles! (If you *do* lose 25 pounds or drop four dress sizes, do let me know. My address is PO Box 618, Coulsdon, Surrey CR5 1RU.)

THE DIET

How long is it since you experimented with your diet? Are you stuck in the same old rut of toast for breakfast, sandwiches for lunch, and meat with two vegetables for dinner? Do you fill the odd hunger gap with chocolate or sweets? Do you drink over the recommended alcohol limit each week (14 units for women, 21 for men – 1 unit is half a pint of beer, one glass of wine or one 'short' drink)? Do you frequently go on slimming diets, then put all the weight back on again?

If you eat an unimaginative diet which is heavy on fatty foods, contains quite a lot of alcohol, and is also fairly high in sugar, then you are not doing your looks and health justice. This is not the place to lecture you on the dangers of a bad diet. Instead, let's consider the advantages of a good one.

By a 'good' diet, I mean one that includes a wide variety of foods which actively help to maintain your body in tip-top condition. Most people eat such a limited range of foods that they have no idea how much better you can feel, and look, simply by ringing the changes. The New You eating programme is delicious, and the recipes are simple and inexpensive to prepare.

During the next 30 days, you will feast on a marvellous range of goodies including the following:

Vitamins A, C and E otherwise known as the 'antioxidant' vitamins that help to protect your body from 'free radicals', which contribute to ageing, and the degeneration of skin, body, and good health. They are in fruits and vegetables – and we simply don't get enough of them!

Whole Grains like wholewheat cereals and rice, and wholemeal bread, which supply Vitamins B and E, to help beat stress and keep your skin looking good. Grains are rich in fibre too, to help regulate your body, and beat sluggishness.

Protein foods like lean meat, pulses and fish. These are the body-builders which help repair and maintain your body in good shape.

Water to 'flush' your body, keep things regular and help improve your skin.

The diet is light on milk and cheese, which can cause fluid retention in many people. However, there is plenty of calcium, in leafy greens and yogurt, for healthy bones and teeth.

Caffeine is cut drastically. If you find that you experience some 'withdrawal' symptoms when deprived of your coffee, don't worry – a slight headache for a day or so is quite normal. However, it is a good idea to persevere if you can.

Every day, you will find that there is a set breakfast menu, a lunch and supper, plus between-meals snacks. Don't try to speed up weight loss by cutting out the snacks; it will not work. You may find that you feel very full after each meal. This is because there are fewer refined foods and more natural foods than you have been used to. Natural foods are far more satisfying and give your brain those useful 'full up' signals.

HOW TO SHOP I recommend that you read through the first seven days of the programme carefully and make a shopping list. Buy all the non-perishable and 'dry' produce you need in one go at your local supermarket. Shop for the perishable produce such as fruit and vegetables every day or two, to ensure perfect freshness. As you will be eating a lot of fresh food, you may find it is cheaper to buy from a market stall. Do check that the salesman gives you the choicest tomatoes or peaches!

MAKE EACH MEAL SPECIAL So that you enjoy your programme fully, make mealtimes fun. If you have children, you'll find that they love the breakfast dishes, and will enjoy the lunches and suppers too. Encourage the rest of your family to join in, adding extra jacket potatoes, baked beans or other vegetables to satisfy man-sized appetites.

IF YOU ARE A MALE 'NEW YOU' Men who wish to follow the programme should add two extra slices of wholemeal bread or a 7oz (200g) jacket potato daily. They should also increase the protein allowance slightly, by adding extra meat or fish. If you are in a strenuous job, you will also need additional complex carbohydrates, such as cereal and vegetables. If in doubt, consult your doctor.

THE EXERCISES
The exercises on the New You programme are divided into four sections: Breathing, Posture, Problem Area and Facial exercises.

Every day, you will be required to perform the Complete Breath breathing exercise and the Complete Posture programme. In addition, you will choose 'Problem Area' exercises (which are carefully structured to avoid straining) to help smooth out your own particular 'wobbly' bits. The facial exercises are recommended for everyone, as they do give a tremendous 'lift' to the whole facial area. In fact, they worked so well for one of our volunteers, Michelle Gibson, that she was accused of paying a sneaky visit to a cosmetic surgeon during the 30-day programme.

COMPLETE BREATH This is a terrific exercise to do in the garden or in front of an open window. It wakes you up, so it is great in the morning, or after a day spent huddled over a hot stove or office desk. Based on a yoga movement, it encourages you to make full use of your lungs – for a change!

1. Stand with your back straight, head erect and legs and feet together, with hands hanging loosely by your sides.

2. Now, inhale deeply, at the same time bringing your arms slowly up at the sides, with palms uppermost.

3. Let the backs of your hands touch above your head.

4. Exhale as you lower your arms back down to your sides. Don't rush – just let the air come out through your mouth very gently.

5. Repeat 6–8 times.

COMPLETE POSTURE PROGRAMME If you stand well, you can look 5 pounds thinner immediately. The trouble is that most of us hunch our shoulders, stick out our tums and bums and look a mess.

During the 30-day programme, you are going to relearn the art of standing and walking gracefully. You will probably 'grow' a few centimetres, and you will certainly feel a lot better.

Ideally, your body should be stretched upwards so that your backbone is in its natural curve but not held stiffly. Your weight should be evenly balanced on both feet, hip girdle held evenly, both hips on the same level. Buttock muscles should be constantly contracted slightly, tummy held in, shoulders kept down and back a little (but never forced back), arms held loosely by your sides. If an imaginary straight line was drawn from your ear to the ground, it would pass through your neck, shoulder joint, elbow, hand, hip, knee and the front of your ankle.

Correct posture has so many health benefits that it is a shame that a large number of us spend our lives slouched over the television, cramped up in cars or heaving shopping bags around. If you stand well, you will feel less tired at the end of the day, your organs will be less cramped, lungs able to expand fully, food will be digested better, and you will be less likely to get arthritis later in life. One of the less well-known consequences of bad posture is that the body will often try to correct the balance itself by building up flab in funny places – on thighs, in pads around the tummy and hips and even around the ankles.

So, do this exercise routine, in front of a long mirror if possible, *every* single day. As well as improving your posture, it also gives you an excellent warm-up before the spot-reducing exercises which will tackle your personal problem areas.

1. *Pelvic Lift* Stand, sideways on to the mirror with your feet slightly apart. Now raise your arms above your head. Exhale as you pull in your tummy muscles, contract your buttocks, and raise your pubic bone so your pelvis is tilted forwards and upwards. Now, raise your breastbone to elongate your ribcage, giving maximum room for breathing. Inhale. Stand in this position for a count of four, breathing normally, then exhale slowly as you lower your arms.

You will notice how much slimmer you appear already. Try to remember the Pelvic Lift position – correcting your posture when your are standing or walking. Tuck in those wobbly bits and they'll (almost!) disappear.

2. *Leg and Arm Spine Stretch* Stand straight, feet together, hands by your sides. (Remember that Pelvic Lift position!) Now, step back with your left foot, keeping your weight forward, left heel off the ground. Raise your right arm above your head. Raise your left leg and push your right arm back, still keeping your right leg straight. Repeat 6 times with left leg, right arm, then 6 with right leg, left arm.

3. *Curved Arm Side Bends* Stand straight, feet about 2 feet apart, hands by your sides. Now raise your right arm above your head and bend your body, from the waist only, over to the left as far as you can go. Straighten up and repeat to the right. Do 6 bends each way.

4. *Split Lunges* Stand with both feet on the floor, hands on your hips, right leg straight out in front, left leg straight out behind, legs wide apart. Now, bend your right knee, moving the weight onto it. Keep your back straight and get as low as you can without leaning forward. Repeat 6 times.

5. *Squats* Stand with feet about 2 feet apart, back straight, hands behind your head. Make sure your feet are facing slightly outwards. Now, keeping your back perfectly straight, squat down. Do not lean forwards – just go as far as you can. Straighten up slowly. Repeat 5 times.

6. *Trunk Twists* Stand straight, feet about 3 feet apart, hands up at shoulder level, fingers tightly clasped in front of you. (Remember that Pelvic Lift posture!) Now, keeping your body straight, feet straight, raising the right heel, twist to the left as far as possible, round to the front, then to the right. Repeat 6 times.

WIND DOWN EXERCISE Repeat this exercise after each exercise session – whether you are simply doing the posture routine or a full set of 'problem' area exercises as well.

Lie on your back on the floor, feet slightly apart, hands by your sides with palms uppermost. Push your back into the floor, and pull in your tummy, tilting your pelvis upwards (this is the lying-down version of the Pelvic Lift exercise). Let your feet flop open and relax, breathing evenly. Now stretch your right arm above your head, right leg down pointing the toe hard. Repeat twice, then repeat with your left arm and leg. Relax for a few moments, then stand up slowly.

PROBLEM AREAS You can make a real impact on those problem areas in 30 days. But do not rush and strain your muscles. Instead, follow each set of exercises, stage by stage. Go on to the more difficult stage only where indicated on your programme. If it seems too difficult, go back to the first stage once more. Never strain yourself. If you have a history of back trouble or any physical injury which could make exercising risky, do consult your doctor before trying these, or any other, exercises.

TUMMY
Stage One
1. Lie on your back, knees bent, feet flat on the floor, hands resting lightly on your tummy.

2. Exhale, pushing the air out of your mouth and pulling in your tummy at the same time. Rock slightly backwards on your bottom so your pelvis is tilted upwards. Breath easily, holding that position and keeping your tummy in.

3. Place your hands behind your head, and – exhaling – raise your knees. At the same time, press upwards with your hands so your head and shoulders are lifted off the floor. Hold the position, briefly, then relax down to the starting position. Repeat 5 times, increasing to 10.

Stage Two

1. Go into the position you learned in Stage One, relax for a few minutes, holding in your tummy, pelvis tilted upwards.

2. Repeat the whole of Stage One, and relax.

3. Now place your hands behind your head and exhale as you lift your head and knees, bending forwards and aiming your right elbow at your left knee. Relax, breathing normally, and then repeat, this time aiming your left elbow at your right knee. Repeat 5 times.

Stage Three

1. Repeat Stages One and Two. Now go back to the first position, knees bent and slightly apart. Place your hands on the backs of your thighs, just below knee level.

2. Exhale and raise your upper body off the ground (using your tummy muscles *not* your back – by now, you should know where they are!), rounding your back slightly.

3. Release your hands and thrust them through your legs for a count of five, then relax back, breathing normally. Repeat 5 times.

Stage Four

1. Repeat Stages One, Two and Three. Now go back to the first position, and relax for a few moments. Place your hands flat on the floor beside you, palms down.

2. Raise your legs off the ground to the vertical position, knees slightly bent, ankles crossed. Pull in your tummy and tilt your pelvis upwards. Now, your bottom and lower back should be off the floor. Place your hands behind your head and raise your chest off the floor. Hold briefly, then relax. Repeat 10 times.

Stage Five
1. Repeat Stages One, Two, Three and Four.

2. Now raise your head slightly, pull in your tummy, lift your feet off the floor and 'cycle'. Make sure your legs are low – not high in the air. Breathe regularly throughout for a count of ten.

BOTTOM, HIPS AND THIGHS
Stage One
1. Lie on the floor on your tummy, hands on the floor under your chin, palms down.

2. Now press down with your hands as you raise your left leg as high as you can. Cross it over your right leg, lower to touch the floor, raise and then lower to starting position.

3. Repeat with right leg.

4. Repeat the whole movement 10 times.

Stage Two
1. Repeat Stage One, relax for moment, then roll over onto your back.

2. Lie with your knees bent, feet flat on the floor, feet shoulders' width apart, hands by your sides, palms down.

3. Squeeze your buttock muscles together and gently raise your hips off the floor. Keep squeezing and

gently lifting, repeat 10 times, without relaxing between lifts. Make sure your back is close to the floor at all times.

Stage Three
1. Repeat Stages One and Two, relax for a few moments, still lying on your back.

2. Now, with hands by your sides, palms down, raise your legs so that your knees and feet are directly above your hips.

3. Open your legs as wide as possible, point your toes towards you and bring your legs together, resisting your own body weight as you do so. Repeat 10 times.

Stage Four
1. Repeat Stages One, Two and Three, relax for a few moments, then roll over onto your left side.

2. Bend your left knee slightly, place your right hand on the floor in front of you for balance, place your left elbow on the floor and lean your head on your left hand.

3. Now stretch your right leg out to the side and slightly back, keeping your foot parallel to the floor. Lift your right leg towards the ceiling and lower slowly. Repeat 10 times, without relaxing between lifts.
4. Change sides and repeat.

Stage Five
1. Repeat Stages One, Two, Three and Four, lie down and relax for a few moments.

2. Sit up carefully. Bend your right knee and clasp it with both hands, pulling it well into your chest, foot flat on the floor. Now gently raise and lower your left leg

10 times without letting it rest on the floor between movements.

3. Change legs and repeat.

WAIST AND MIDRIFF
Stage One
1. Stand with your legs apart, hands behind your head, elbows out to the side (don't forget your Pelvic Lift!).

2. Now bend your torso from left to right without twisting your body. Repeat 10 times each side.

Stage Two
1. Repeat Stage One. Now stand with feet apart holding a large can of baked beans or tomatoes in each hand.

2. Raise your arms to shoulder level and bend your elbows.

3. Punch your right hand hard to the right, twisting round to the right with your torso (keep your hips facing the front), as far as you can.

4. Return to the first position, and punch your left fist to the left, again twisting your body round as far as possible.

BUST
Stage One
1. Stand or sit with your arms up at chest level, elbows bent.

2. Now clasp your right wrist with your left hand, left wrist with your right hand.

3. Push hands sharply towards your elbows, 50 times. You should see your bosom 'jump' slightly if you are doing it correctly.

Stage Two

1. Repeat Stage One. Stand straight, feet slightly apart, holding a large can of baked beans or tomatoes in each hand.

2. Raise hands to shoulder height, palms facing inwards. Raise your hands right up above your head, pause briefly, then lower them slowly. Repeat 10 times, increasing to 15.

Stage Three

1. Repeat Stages One and Two. Now lie across your bed on your back holding one can with both hands.

2. Position yourself so your head is hanging over the side of the bed, but make sure your neck is adequately supported.

3. Now raise your arms straight above your chest. Hold the position briefly, and lower the can behind your head, keeping your arms straight and allowing them to go as low as possible using their own weight as leverage.

4. Hold briefly then raise the weight above your head once more. Repeat 10 times, increasing to 25 or 30.

SHOULDERS
Stage One

1. Sit on a chair, clasping your hands loosely behind your back, elbows slightly bent.

2. Draw the shoulder blades together, at the same time, press your upper arms towards each other across your back. Don't straighten you elbows. Hold briefly, then rest.

3. Repeat 6 times.

Stage Two

1. Repeat Stage One. Now clasp your hands in front of you, and sit with your back straight, shoulders relaxed.

2. Raise your clasped hands above your head, without pushing it forward.

3. Lower your clasped hands behind your neck – again making sure that your head doesn't go forward. Hold briefly, return to position 2 and then position 1 in this exercise.

4. Repeat 6 times.

Stage Three

1. Repeat Stages One and Two. Now, stand with your feet about 10 inches apart, holding a can of tomatoes or baked beans in each hand. Your arms should be straight down with your palms facing your thighs.

2. Now raise your right arm over your head. Lower it slowly, at the same time raising your left arm. Make the movement steady, moving the arms simultaneously with the cans passing each other at shoulder height.

3. Repeat 10 times with each arm.

BACK

Stage One

1. Lie on your tummy on the floor, hands with palms flat on the floor at shoulder level.

2. Straighten your arms to raise the top half of your body only off the floor. Look up at the ceiling, feeling your spine curve.

3. Lower your body slowly. Repeat 5 times.

Stage Two

1. Repeat Stage One. Kneel on the floor and place your hands on the floor in front of you with hands shoulders' width apart. Knees should be together, feet stretched out (do not push your toes into the floor).

2. Now hollow your back, head up. Hold for a count of five.

3. Slowly, arch your back, letting your head hang down. Count five. Repeat the whole exercise 5 times.

RESTING BACK POSITION

This is a useful 'exercise' for back relief. But do check with your doctor or physiotherapist if in any doubt.

1. Place a large bolster or two pillows, one on top of each other, on the floor, with a couple of smaller cushions for head support.

2. Lie down with your shoulders on the bolster, head hanging back over the edge of the bolster, supported by the cushions.

3. Now lie back and breathe deeply. Raise your arms over your head and stretch up your fingers.

4. Hold the position for a few moments, then lower your arms and relax.

5. Gently, roll over on your side and get up onto your hands and knees, sit back on your heels for a few seconds, then stand up.

FACIAL EXERCISES These are for relaxation, and to help tone up facial muscles.

DOUBLE CHIN

1. Let your head hang back. Contract the muscles in the front of your neck.

2. Close teeth tightly. Clench your jaws until the chords of your neck stand out. Open and close jaws 6 times.

3. Now lower your chin, jaws still clenched.

4 Turn your head to the left and the right, 4 times each. Relax.

CHUBBY CHEEKS

1. Place your hands on the sides of your face. Gently push upward, so the crow's feet under your eyes are smoothed away.

2. Pull outward, so you smooth out your chubby cheeks.

3. Push your lips forward, and say 'O'.

4. Point your lips to the left and to the right. You will feel a strong pull on your cheek muscles as you do this. Repeat 10 times each side.

PUFFY EYES

1. Place the tip of the third finger of each hand in the hollow at the sides of your face, just beside each eye. Press firmly but gently.

2. Blink 10 times, then close eyes and relax.

3. Open eyes wide, and focus on a distant object. Hold for a count of five.

WALKING PROGRAMME You will lose weight and shape up more quickly if you walk every single day throughout the 30 days. Walking is probably the most underestimated form of exercise. In terms of health benefits, you really cannot beat it. Walking helps rev up your heart, improves your lung capacity, exercises every part of your body. Calorie expenditure during walking is quite significant, too. For instance, if you walk on level ground for half an hour at around 2mph, you will burn off approximately 90 calories. If you step up your rate to, say, 3mph, the calorie burn-up increases to 130, the equivalent of a small chocolate bar. That might not sound very much, but the effect of a brisk walk on your metabolic rate continues after you stop – giving additional calorie-burning power. Not bad for a form of keeping fit which is natural, easy, and most important, free!

Now try stepping out. You should start off with ten minutes of easy walking, warming up to a much more brisk pace, then easing down again. Never, ever walk briskly to start with – your muscles are cold and you could strain them.

Style Please adopt a good posture (do the Complete Posture programme exercises before you set off if you can. They will warm you up and establish correct posture before you start). Your walking style should be easy and relaxed. Do not carry shopping (have your shoulder bag slung across your body for good balance), walk with your arms swinging comfortably but not exaggeratedly and your toes pointing forward. If you walk with your toes pointing inwards, your whole body frame has to adjust to cope and you could develop hard skin on your feet, and cause poor circulation.

Wear comfortable walking shoes or trainers and socks, a loose tracksuit or leggings. No jeans!

On your 30-day programme I have given you a target to aim for each day. If you can do more . . . great!

Stage One Walk for 20 minutes – 10 minutes easy, 5 minutes brisk, 5 minutes easy.

Stage Two Walk for 30 minutes – 10 minutes easy, 15 minutes brisk, 5 minutes easy.

Stage Three Walk for 45 minutes – 10 minutes easy, 20 minutes brisk, 15 minutes easy.

When you are walking, the simplest way to establish a rhythm is to count your paces over a period of 10 seconds, then multiply by 60 to work out your speed. For instance, a speed of 3mph is 88 paces per minute. That speed is 'brisk'.

But take care: If you feel tired, stop. Take your pulse. If, after 10 minutes' rest, your heart is still beating over 100 beats per minute, take things more slowly. Never walk in great heat or cold, or when it is pouring down with rain. Never flop down motionless after your walk. Rest, certainly, but move your arms and legs about to keep your circulation brisk until your heart rate returns to normal.

(For Foot Exercises *see* Treats For Your Feet on page 33.)

CHAPTER THREE

YOUR PERSONAL BEAUTY PLAN

When time is short and money is tight, the first thing to suffer is your beauty routine. Shame! On our New You programme, you will learn to spend a little time and effort on yourself. Around half an hour a day is all you need. That's not much but the results will be truly spectacular.

You will start the programme with beauty baths, hair and facial treatments. Later, when your skin and hair are beginning to feel the benefit of the diet and exercise plan, you will be able to try out the hair styling and make-up tips from experts Joshua Galvin and Jan Wright. Once a week, take time out for a manicure, pedicure and body massage. The routines I explain below are very simple.

BEAUTY BATHS

Every day, throughout the 30 days, you *must* treat yourself to one of these beauty baths. Pick the ones that will help your own particular skin best. All ingredients are available from health food shops, chemists or specialist beauty shops like Body Shop.

1. *Anti-Cellulite Scrub* In a screwtop jar, mix together 2 teaspoons (10ml) of grapeseed oil, 5 drops juniper essential oil, 2 drops lemon essential oil. Pour the mixture over 3oz (75g) polenta or cornmeal (available from

supermarkets). It will form a gritty paste. Rub this firmly into damp skin on your hips, bottom and thighs. Do it really thoroughly, using circular movements upwards. You could use a rough flannel or mitt for your massage. Then shower off all the gritty bits. Try this four times a week if you have persistent cellulite.

2. *Perfumed Bath* Add 2 teaspoons (10ml) of olive or sunflower oil to your bath, plus 3 or 4 drops of rose or jasmine essential oil. Both are delicious scents which will make you feel luxurious and pampered. Wallow!

3. *Moisturizing Bath* If your skin is dry, fill cotton sachets (or cut up old handkerchiefs and make them into sachets) with finely ground oatmeal and place in the bath while the water is running. Once you are in the tub, scrub away dead, dingy skin with the sachet. This is just great to smooth away that dead skin from your elbows, ankles, and bottom!

4. *Stimulating Bath* If you feel very tired and have to go out, add dried peppermint or mint leaves to your bath water. Simply put them inside a cotton sachet and place under the running water.

Other envigorating baths are those with essential oils such as lemon, mandarin, jasmine and peppermint. These are great if you have to make an early start, too.

5. *Relaxing Bath* Add two camomile teabags to the water to help relax muscles. Or, a few drops of lavender oil will do the same job.

FACE TREATMENTS

You do not have to spend a fortune on expensive products to have healthy, glowing skin. Try one of these treatments twice a week during your 30-day make-over. (*See* also page 38.)

1. *Moisturizing Masks* Mix together half a small avo-cado, one egg yolk, 1 teaspoon (5ml) of olive oil to make a gooey cream. Plaster it onto clean skin – all over your throat, neck and upper chest as well as the dry bits on your face. (Make sure your hair is out of the way.) Relax for 15 minutes, then remove with damp cotton wool.

Or, mash an overripe banana with a spoonful of cream, milk or yogurt, add a little honey (and an egg yolk if your skin is very dry). Use as above.

2. *Complexion Booster* If your skin looks grey and dingy try this. Mix together 1oz (25g) brewer's yeast powder, 4 tablespoons (60ml) of fresh apple juice and 2 tablespoons (30ml) of plain yogurt. Dissolve the yeast powder in the apple juice, stir in the yogurt and apply as above. You'll need to apply a moisturizer after this one.

3. *Skin Refiner* This is good if your skin is 'muddy'. Mix 1oz (25g) ground almonds with 1 tablespoon (15ml) of runny honey and one lightly beaten egg white. Apply as above. Before you rinse the mixture off, massage it well into the areas around your nose and chin where debris often collects. Rinse thoroughly and moisturize.

4. *Oily Skin Masks* Try mashing 1 tablespoon (15ml) of softened melon flesh with a little natural yogurt. Beat an egg white and fold into the mixture. Leave on your skin for 15 minutes, then rinse with tepid water.

Or, make washing grains by mixing a little cold water with a handful of ordinary porridge oats and rub the mixture onto your face, paying particular attention to blackheads and oily patches.

MANICURE AND PEDICURE

Try these two very simple, step-by-step routines once a week. (Remember that you should always file your nails *before* a bath and not after, as nails become very soft after soaking in hot water.)

HANDS

1. You need cotton wool, nail varnish remover, orange sticks, emery boards, hand cream, cuticle remover, base coat, nail varnish and top coat. Start by removing old varnish: hold cotton wool between first and second fingers and rub nails against it rather than the other way around.

2. Now file nails gently away from you; make an smooth oval shape and don't file away too much nail at the side, or the nails will snap more easily and could develop hang-nails and soreness. Emery boards are less harsh than metal nail files.

3. Use the pointed end of an orange stick plus a small piece of cotton wool to clean away any dirt or debris under the nail. A little cuticle remover on the cotton wool will help clean the area thoroughly.

4. Apply tiny blobs of cuticle remover or cream to each cuticle. Smooth in very gently. Now, using the wedge-end of the orange stick, ease back the cuticle and remove any stray bits of skin which come away until the half-moon (which is really the top of the matrix or growth area of the nail) is revealed.

5. Apply a little extra nail varnish remover to each nail to get rid of greasiness before the varnish is applied. Using base coat and painting the nails on your right hand first, make three strokes on each nail: centre, left

side, then right side, working from the half-moon to the tip.

6. Allow nails 10 minutes to dry before applying top coat. Dark enamels usually need only two coats, lighter shades require three. Apply a top coat of clear gloss for extra shine and protection.

FEET

1. You need two old towels, tissues, cotton wool, nail varnish and remover, orange sticks, nail scissors, emery boards, and body lotion.

2. Place one towel on a chair and the other on the floor in front of it. Place a tissue on the towel and put your foot on this. Remove old nail enamel carefully by holding cotton wool between first and second fingers and rubbing gently against toe-nails, so remover does not touch the enamel on your fingers.

3. Rub body lotion generously into your foot and around the toe-nails. Spend a little time thoroughly rubbing the cream in, work it between the toes, and around the heel. Place your foot on the towel on the floor while you deal with the other one.

4. Working on the first foot again, remove grime and dry bits from behind the nails and around cuticles with an orange stick. Work gently.

5. Now cut nails straight across (don't round them at the corners – this encourages ingrowing toe-nails), and file away any rough bits.

6. Apply polish remover again to remove all traces of grease from nails. Separate toes with wads of cotton wool. Apply polish with three decisive strokes per nail,

centre, left and right. Repeat with the other foot. Walk around the house or sit and watch television barefoot for 10 minutes before applying second coat.

Once a month Give your feet the full treatment by using cuticle remover to get rid of ragged bits of cuticle and hard skin. Clip it away with clippers but make sure you don't snip any living tissue.

TREATS FOR YOUR FEET
Try these cheap and cheerful foot treatment.

Foot Refresher After shopping, your daily walk, or working on your feet all day, dabble your toes in a bowl of luke-warm water with 1 tablespoon (15ml) of cider vinegar or lemon juice. Cider vinegar is particularly good if you have itchy toes after wearing trainers for long periods.

Hard Skin treatment Mix 2 tablespoons (30ml) of ordinary cooking oil with 6 drops of lavender essence and heat gently in a pan until warm but not too hot. Rub into your feet, put on pair of old socks and sleep in them. If you are feeling flush, almond oil is even better.

FOOT EXERCISES Try these:
1. Sit on a chair, legs straight out in front. Point toes to the ceiling, then straight ahead, alternately. Now rotate feet clockwise, then anti-clockwise.

2. Drop a pencil on the floor and try to pick it up using bare feet.

3. Stand straight, rise up on tiptoe, hold the position briefly, then lower. Repeat rapidly, then try it with one foot at a time.

4. During your 30-day programme, try to walk barefoot in the house as much as possible, if you have smooth flooring or fitted carpets. Avoid soft slippers but keep a comfy, well-made pair at home to change into.

MASSAGE

This do-it-yourself massage is very simple and relaxing. Try it where indicated on your 30-day programme. (Of course, if you have a partner who is prepared to do this for you, great!)

1. You need a warm room with sufficient space to lie down, a large towel, body lotion or oil (use one of the recipes below if you wish), and tissues. Lie down on the towel on your back and relax for a moment. Pour a little lotion or oil on your tummy and rub it with circular movements.

2. Roll over. Press your fingertips on either side of your spine and rub gently. Bring your hands above shoulder level and rub shoulder blades, neck and shoulders in stroking movements.

3. Sit up slowly, take some more lotion and kneed and press your legs. Work from the thighs towards the knees, then back again. Now work from the knees down to the ankles, and back again.

4. Still sitting, press the tips of your thumbs either side of your spine. Press for a few seconds, relax and move your thumbs up and down about an inch. Repeat, working up as far as you can. Now stand up and pinch your buttocks! If you have cellulite, kneed away at the fatty bits, pinching lightly.

5. Cover a chair with your towel, sit on it and work lotion into your feet. The easiest way to do this is to rest one foot on the opposite thigh (like a modified 'half lotus' yoga position), and work really hard with fingers and thumbs all over the sole of your foot and between your toes. Repeat with the other foot.

6. Now blot off the surplus oil, put on a bathrobe and rest for as long as you can. If possible, put on an old tracksuit to allow the massage lotion to sink into your body. If you have to go out, have a quick shower to whisk away any surplus oil.

MASSAGE OILS You can turn your massage session into a relaxing or an envigorating beauty treatment if you add a few drops of essential oil to a base of ordinary cooking oil. You can buy essential oils at health food shops and Body Shop branches. A small bottle goes a very long way, as you need very little. Add oil to your bath water too.

Here are some suggestions: Neroli Oil is warming, relaxing and calming; Mandarin Oil peps you up after a busy day; Jasmine lifts depression and stress and is very good if you have menstrual cramps; Lavender is fortifying, and a good choice if you have a hectic evening ahead.

YOUR HAIR

As the month progresses, you will feel more vigorous and ready for change. If you need a new hair-do, I recommend waiting until the third week of the programme before you make any decisions. Our guinea-pigs were all dissatisfied with their hair, but I persuaded them to wait until they had lost a few pounds and were feeling more confident before taking the plunge!

While they were waiting, they tried out these easy hair treatments to help get their hair in the best possible condition before that trim, perm or colour treatment:

Hot Oil treatment for dry hair Heat 2 tablespoons (30 ml) of olive or corn oil, saturate your hair and cover with a plastic bag or shower cap. Add heat with a heavy towel or by aiming a hair dryer at your head. Leave for 10 minutes, then shampoo in the normal way.

Protein treatment for brittle hair with split ends Beat together one egg, 1 tablespoon (15 ml) of castor, olive or corn oil and 1 teaspoon (5 ml) cider vinegar. Shampoo hair once, apply the mixture, wrap in a towel or pop on a shower cap and leave for 15 minutes. Rinse, shampoo lightly and condition.

Scalp Exercises Curl up each hand as though you were grasping a tennis ball, with your fingers tensed. Press the 'cushion' of each finger on your scalp with a circular motion until you feel the warmth of blood flowing to your scalp. Then move on to another area, until your whole scalp is tingling.

HOW TO CHOOSE A NEW STYLE A new hairstyle can be the most uplifting beauty treat of all – or the most disastrous.

Follow these rules from top hair stylist Joshua Galvin who created all the new styles for our volunteers:

1. Take a long look at yourself in a full-length mirror. Does your hair balance your body? Is it too long, dragging you down? Is it too short, giving a pinhead effect? If you have a big frame, you need soft, voluminous hair, mid-length but not too long. Large people who surround

themselves with masses of hair, just make their faces look smaller and their bodies bigger.

If you are short and plump, too much hair will be overwhelming. You need a fair amount of volume, and some lift. A chignon will make your neckline look longer. Avoid dramatic cuts, which can look too harsh.

2. Now take your hair back from your face. If you have a wide forehead, narrow chin and small cheekbones, don't wear your hair past your shoulders as it will emphasize the narrowness of your chin. Ponytails are out. Go for a hairstyle with forward movement such as a bob.

If you have a square face, you need to soften it with hair that falls onto the face in curls or waves, or is swept off to the side. If you face is plump, you need a little more hair around it to make it appear smaller.

3. Now study your features. If you have a double chin, avoid short shapes and go for a medium length, below ear level. Cover ears that stick out, and never swamp a short neck with a mass of hair. If you have a high forehead, don't be tempted to cover it with a long, straight fringe. Instead, go for softer, lighter tendrils. Big nose? Don't tie your hair back – choose a soft style with hair falling forward to reduce the impact of your nose.

4. When you have looked at yourself carefully, think about the practical side. Your new style must fit in with your lifestyle, and it must also be suitable for your hair type. For instance, if you work outside it is no good choosing a long, wavy hair-do if you have thin, wispy hair that will not hold a curl. You are either going to have to have a perm (which may not be suitable for your hair), or be continually setting it on heated rollers which will make it even whispier! Study magazine pictures of

the type of style you have in mind, cut out some suitable ones and take them along to your hairdresser.

5. Book a consultation (free, or it should be) with the hairdresser before you finally choose your style. Chat at length about your likes and dislikes (do not be persuaded to have something that you don't like) and discuss exactly how much it is all going to cost. Make sure you talk about how you can keep up the style yourself between salon visits. Never go for a radical, all-over colour change which will need three-weekly re-growth attention. Instead, ask for a colour conditioner, highlights or low lights for a subtler effect. Consider, too, the versatility of the style. If you play sport, you may want a style which you wash and let dry naturally, but which can also be set into a smoother shape with heated rollers when you are working.

SKIN CARE AND MAKE-UP
You will be delighted to find that your skin improves dramatically during your 30-day New You programme. All our volunteers were thrilled when they noticed their skins became clearer and softer, thanks to the diet and exercise programme.

Wait until the third week to try out Jan Wright's great make-up tips below, but make time for one of these easy skin treatments once or twice a week throughout the programme. They are all cheap, using every-day ingredients from your larder:

GREASY SKIN
Tomato Mask Mash a squashed tomato to a pulp, blend with 1 dessertspoon (10 ml) of natural, unsweetened

yogurt and apply to clean skin. Leave for 15 minutes, then wash off carefully with tepid water.

Brewers Yeast Facial Make a stiff paste with 1 table-spoon (15ml) of brewer's yeast flakes or powder, a little milk or yogurt, and a dash of rose water. Plaster onto your skin, leave for 10 minutes, then wash off with tepid water and apply a non-alcohol toner.

Cucumber Mask Put a quarter of a cucumber into a blender, give it a whirl, and blend in a stiffly beaten egg white and a dash of peppermint essence. Plaster the mask onto clean skin, leave for 15 minutes, and rinse.

DRY SKIN
Peach Facial Select a squashy peach, peel and remove stone, and mash the flesh with 1 teaspoon (5ml) honey and a little milk. Plaster onto clean skin, lie down for 15 minutes, then remove with tissues. This leaves your skin feeling lovely and soft.

Banana Pack Mash one small ripe banana in a bowl, add 1 tablespoon (15ml) of finely ground oatmeal and 1 teaspoon (5ml) runny honey. Stir well, apply to clean face and neck, relax for 20 minutes and remove with warm water. Apply your favourite moisturizing cream afterwards.

COMBINATION SKIN
Apple and Oatmeal Mask Mix together 1 tablespoon (15ml) of ground oatmeal, 1 tablespoon (15ml) of nat-ural unsweetened yogurt, half a freshly grated apple, and 2 teaspoons (10ml) of lemon juice. Apply to clean skin, relax for 20 minutes and remove with warm water.

MAKE-UP TIPS TO CHANGE YOUR IMAGE Here's a secret: in real life, the model-girl beauties in the magazines look *nothing* like their pictures. The glamorous image is always down to the work of a brilliant make-up artist. In fact, the blanker and more boring the model's face is, the better. For then, the make-up artist can use it, just like the canvas of a painting, to create any look he or she desires.

Your face isn't model-girl blank, it's full of character. Yes, that huge nose, those awful freckles, that crooked chin – they are all great. The only problem is that most of us would rather look like a model! You can do just that by following this very simple make-up routine devised by Jan Wright. She used Rimmel cosmetics throughout, which proves that you do not need to spend large amounts of money to look sensational. See the results of her work in the colour plate section, with full details of the products she used.

Easy Make-Up

1. Start by preparing your 'canvas'. Smooth a light moisturizer all over your face and neck and let it sink in for a few moments.

2. Apply a light, beige-tinted foundation with a dampened cosmetic sponge, in downward strokes to smooth out the hairs on your face. Take it down under your chin, and blend into your neck.

3. Apply loose powder with a clean brush or cotton wool, pressing into the skin, then brushing off the surplus with a fresh brush or cottonwool.

4. Use a tawny or peachy blusher with a very light touch and a large brush to shade your face. Soften the corners of a square face with blusher on lower cheeks

and temples. Give a round face interesting angles by using it on your cheeks in upwards strokes towards ear-level. A little dark shading under your chin and around your jawline will shorten an oblong face and you can 'plump out' the cheeks of a pear-shaped face with a rosier shade. Use more tawny shader to soften the temples and prevent a triangular look from spoiling a good shape. Make sure all edges are blended in, and double check by looking at your profile in the mirror.

5. Brush brows upwards into a neat line and pluck out any stragglers underneath, stretching the skin with the first and second fingers of the left hand while you pluck with the tweezers held firmly in the right. To check where the brow line should end, hold your eyebrow pencil against your nose so it makes a line through the outer corner of your eye to your brow. Carefully, brush brows towards your nose, pencil in light feathery strokes to correct and darken the brow, then brush brows upwards and outwards to cover the strokes. Colour with a greyish brown or soft brown pencil only, never black.

6. To make the most of your eyes, follow these tips. First use a creamy concealer all over the eye area. If it comes in a stick, apply it with a brush, to minimize dragging the skin on this delicate area. Select soft colours – browns, beiges and pinky-peach colours are flattering on most people. If your eyes are too close together, make them appear wide apart by using a pale shadow on the inner corners, a 'wing' of darker shadow from the centre lid upwards and outwards, and a little Kohl or soft pencil on the outer corner of the eye only. If your eyes are too wide apart, reverse the process, using darker shadow on the inner corners, shading from the

inner corner outwards, stopping at the natural outer corner of each eye. You can open up too-small eyes with light shadows around the eye, and beigey/brown wings of shadow from socket to brow-bone. If your eyes are hooded, dark shadow will make the lid appear smaller. Blend it into a lighter shadow at the brow-bone. Use more light shadow under the eye area.

.7. Apply eyeliner carefully using an eyeliner wand. Make sure it is very close to the lashes. If you have lids that 'show', you may wish to use a slightly thicker line. Check in the mirror. If you want a more theatrical look for parties, you can flick the line slightly at the corners.

8. Brush mascara upwards on upper lashes, downwards on lower ones. Non-filament mascaras are easier to clean off than the thicker or waterproof ones. When each coat is dry, go over with a clean brush to separate lashes. Up to three coats will give you a lovely, flirty look!

9. Lip shape and colour are a vital part of the fashion look. First, apply foundation on lips. Using a sharp pencil that tones in with your lipstick, trace the outline of your lips. You can correct thin lips slightly by taking the outline just outside your natural shape, and vice versa; but don't overdo it. Nothing looks worse than obviously drawn lips. Now fill in with lip colour, then blot, reapply, and blot again. Top with a little glosser if you want a shiny look. Run your tongue over the inside of your lips, so you can be certain that there will be no trace of lip colour on your teeth.

CHAPTER FOUR

CHANGING YOUR IMAGE

If you become stuck in a rut for a long time, you can get very lazy about your looks and lifestyle. Somehow, it seems simpler to let yourself drift along from day to day wearing the same kind of clothes, cooking the same kind of meals, and doing the same kind of things.

When you look, perhaps enviously, at others, you are convinced that you could never be as dynamic, smart, and interesting as they are. Rubbish! The only person who can control your life is *you*. If you truly *want* to change things, you can.

Our New You volunteers were all women who felt that, somehow, they were not doing themselves justice, either in the way they dressed or the way they projected themselves:

'I had lost confidence after settling down to being a mum,' says Michelle Gibson, age 34. 'Much as I adore looking after my lovely little daughter, Adele, I felt frumpy and boring. I had a wardrobe of glamorous clothes from my working days. Nothing fitted because I'd put on so much weight. I desperately wanted to change.' She did! You can see how much by checking out our pictures in the colour plate section. Even more important than the make-up and hair-styling changes (and the weight-loss – she shed 11 pounds and is still losing) was Michelle's own attitude towards herself. She became far more positive and projected a more glamorous image. She looked far better for it.

Another volunteer, Joy Hawkins, was already holding down a high-powered job as a television researcher when she joined the programme. Joy, age 48, who has a 19-year-old daughter, Beth, felt that her dress-sense didn't really represent the true 'her'. 'I looked like a goody-goody type, whereas I'm rather outgoing and can be a bit wicked at times. Those baggy skirts and tops did nothing for me. Inside, I felt more like a dynamic 'Dynasty' lady than a boring schoolma'm – which is what I looked like.'

During the programme, Joy developed the 'inner' person, and eventually, it took over! She tried some 'power dressing' and found it suited her personality perfectly. Check the results in the black and white plate section.

So, how can you boost your own confidence, and project the image that is really *you*? Amazingly, you can do a great deal to change things in just 30 days. First, you need to do some special 'positive thinking' exercises which will help you to find out more about yourself.

Try at least one of these every day throughout your 30-day programme:

1. Spend 10 minutes each day alone in your sitting-room or bedroom. Put on some relaxing music, take the telephone off the hook. Now lie down on a sofa or the bed, close your eyes and breathe deeply for a few moments. Let your mind wander, with different images flitting in and out of your brain.

Now focus on an image of yourself, looking fit, confident and well-dressed in a familiar situation, perhaps at a party, walking along a favourite beach or entertaining friends at home. You are feeling good, the atmosphere is happy, people are laughing. Keep that image firmly in your mind for a few minutes. Then just relax and let your mind wander again. Every day 'tune in' to that person – he or she is you!

2. Try this variation on the exercise above when things are getting you down. Lie down as before, with some soothing music playing. Imagine yourself, fit and fabulous (of course!), in a beautiful environment such as a lush garden or a sumptuously decorated room. It could be based on your own home, or something you've seen in a magazine or on television. Visualize every detail of the garden or room, from the smallest flower to the luxurious rugs on the floor. This is now your 'sanctuary', somewhere you know you can go back to when things are difficult. Relax, breathing deeply, as you come back to reality.

3. Sit down with a pile of glossy magazines. Go through them, imagining yourself in the gorgeous clothes, looking as sensational as the fashion models. Pick out the things that would look good on you and picture yourself wearing them. Very positive people tend to see themselves as the centre of the universe with everything on it as part of their lives rather than the other way around. This is unhealthy when carried to extremes but a little bit of it does no harm at all. For instance, when a woman like Joan Collins or Stephanie Beacham looks through a magazine the first thing she thinks about is how the outfits would look on her. She flicks through, mentally discarding the clothes or accessories that wouldn't do much for her. Afterwards, she might admire other items but she is number one! I am not advocating that you should suddenly become an insufferable prima donna, just suggesting that a dash of selfishness is not

a bad idea. (I'm not implying that either of the actresses above is a prima donna. I've met Stephanie Beacham once and she is very nice, and I've interviewed Joan three or four times, and she is very 'normal' indeed, but has certainly made positive thinking into an art form!)

4. Go to the cinema and imagine yourself as one of the glamorous, sympathetic characters (*not* a dinosaur!). Picture yourself in the clothes, the situations, the places in the film, cuddling up to the hero. Far fetched? Yes, but just sowing the seeds of possibility in your brain will open up your mind to excitement and adventure, so when they come along, you'll be ready and willing to have fun.

5. Do at least one thing each week that is truly 'for you'. It could be signing on for piano lessons, visiting a museum that you have longed to visit, making love all afternoon, eating breakfast in bed, or just spending half an hour in the bath! Selfish? Not at all. If anyone complains, let them – or tell them this is all part of the New You programme. It is!

6. Every day, try one of these instant Morale Boosters:

a) Wear something pink – pale, deep or 'shocking', whichever suits you best. It is the colour of confidence, warmth, love, affection, fun. If you wear pink, you have a profound effect on others, too. They smile at you (and you smile back!), are more inclined to like your ideas, enjoy your cooking, and even laugh at your jokes.
b) Telephone someone who amuses you. Have a giggle together. You will feel refreshed afterwards.
c) Go for a walk (you *have* to on the programme!).

You will get an extra oxygen boost to your brain, feel better and look better.

d) Chat to someone new. At work, at the bus-stop, at the baby clinic, wherever you happen to be. Pluck up courage to talk to that new person in the office, or the shy assistant in the bank. Brighten someone's day – go on!

CLOTHES FOR CONFIDENCE

Our volunteers all admitted that they loved clothes and looking good, but before the programme most had opted for a 'safe' uniform of baggy skirt and top or (horrors!) black leggings and a voluminous sweatshirt to hide the bulges. Unfortunately, neither of these outfits does a thing for anyone's figure, and certainly does not hide any bulges; both simply accentuate them.

Our guinea-pigs admitted that they knew they had brighter, more interesting clothes hidden away at the back of their wardrobe, but hadn't got the time, energy or inclination to go through them. But, after two weeks on the programme, they were so full of energy that revamping their wardrobes became fun instead of a chore. They have now all found great clothes which they can wear to project a brand new look.

You can do the same. Just follow my plan for clothes confidence:

1. Choose an afternoon when everyone is out, and get everything out of your wardrobe. Arm yourself with a copy of the latest fashion magazine for inspiration. Make one pile of tops and one pile of bottoms. Now experiment by trying on different tops and bottoms together. You are bound to come up with at least three or four fresh-looking outfits which reflect new fashion

trends. For instance, try that old long-line hacking jacket with leggings, boots and a lacy shirt you had forgotten you had. Put together, they are instantly right for this year's fashionable 'dandy' look.

Or, take an old velvet evening jacket (velvet is top fashion again) and team it with jeans and a tight-fitting body, plus some junk jewelry for a trendy party look. If you have got a good-condition black skirt which fits, check the length. You could shorten it, team it with thick black tights and a classic white shirt – you simply need to add a smart jacket or sweater for a great daytime look.

To give you an instant guide to which clothes go together, it is a good idea to hang clothes in your wardrobe in colour sections, with all the navy items together, all the cream items together and so on. It helps if you place a dark colour next to a light one, so the divisions are obvious.

Remember that wire hangers should never be used to hang clothes. They will spoil the shoulders of the garment and could catch on delicate fabrics, ruining your priceless silk shirt or lace evening dress.

Check through shoes and bags, earmark the good ones for repair, and ruthlessly throw out the rest. Go through belts, jewelry, and scarves. The latter are 'in' again, too, so check for gems among your collection which could pull together an outfit.

Now do a little forward planning. Think about the life you are leading, and any imminent outings or holidays; mentally plan just what you will buy as soon as you have some spare cash. Then, your brain will be 'primed' to seek out the right thing as you window-shop. Do not forget the golden rule, which applies whatever your budget may be: spend most money on the 'basics' that will not date – black trousers, a good jacket, a classic sweater. Fun items like gold basques, frilly knickers and silver hot pants should be cheap unless you have a sugar daddy or a large income.

2. Treat yourself to one new item. It could be a waistcoat (Sue Tucker chose hers to complement her trousers, shirts and sweaters – *see* the black and white plate section), or a jacket (Joy Hawkins found a brilliant red number at C & A for just £29.99 which goes with all her black skirts and trousers, and will be great in summer too), or a sweater which will brighten up your whole wardrobe. Make it pink, perhaps?

3. Start wearing your 'best' clothes every day. What are you waiting for? This is not the rehearsal, this is the real thing! Even if you are just going to the shops or to a friend's house for coffee, get dressed up. If you feel depressed or off-colour, dig out the very best thing in your wardrobe and wear it. There is nothing like knowing you are wearing a super outfit to make you feel better instantly.

4. Check out your underwear. Make a note to invest in some new bras, pants and all-in-ones as soon as you can, or make a list of the items you would like for your birthday or for Christmas (it's never too early!). When choosing bras, try on if you possibly can. Be *sure* that you buy a bra in the right size. You may need a larger size but a smaller cup-size. Take a tight-fitting shirt with you, so you can see exactly what it is doing for you (or not doing for you) before you buy it. Do not buy everything in practical black, white or beige. Choose some naughty reds, pinks and blues too, to make you feel wicked.

COLOUR CONFIDENCE

You may have very set ideas about what colours suit you. Perhaps you have always been told that you look beautiful in blue, or that green suits you because you are a red-head. Maybe. However, you should remember that colour is a strong weapon in the image-making game and many colours will suit you (although it may be necessary to pick and choose the exact shade). Use colour to project the image you want and to get the results you want. Here is my guide.

White/Cream Always a good bet if you want to look rich and pampered. White is expensive-looking, cream even better. Great, too, if you are tired – both shades act as a 'reflector', lifting and lightening your face. That is why pearls are so flattering on older women. Take a fresh white T-shirt with you to change into on long aircraft journeys, keep a white or cream skirt as a summer basic, wear a white shirt (pinched from a man, perhaps) with jeans.

Black Not as flattering or as slimming as most women think. If you don't lighten up the effect of a 'little black dress' with glitzy jewelry, you can easily look old and tired. If in doubt, wear black on the bottom half of your body only – a black skirt or trousers with a bright, light jacket *is* a slimming idea for hippy women (and that's most of us!).

Pink/Red Pink is positive in a gentle way, red in a dynamic way. Wear them when you want to make an impact. Good on red-heads, blondes, brunettes, almost everyone, except those with a florid complexion. Soft-pinks look better on blondes, deeper pinks on brunettes. If you are over 40, try the impact of red. Just a touch, such as a bright red sweater, can look great and give you that positive, exciting feeling. There is nothing better for your morale than putting on a gorgeous, cuddly scarlet sweater and jeans or black ski-pants on a dull, boring morning.

Green/Turquoise Cool, relaxing colours which will make you look and feel in control, even in tight situations. Lime is the only difficult shade in the green spectrum, very few people look good in it.

Blue This colour can be downright cold. Think of frosty political ladies decked out in blue, nurses' uniforms, the sea on a winter's day. Wear it when you don't mind being kept at arm's length.

Navy You can't help reminding people of uniforms (policemen, sailors, schoolgirls) when you wear basic navy. This is fine so long as you soften it with beige or pink, or even white. A navy blazer is a great buy. Wear it with jeans, a long pleated skirt, or even shorts. Navy is also wonderful with cream; try a creamy shirt or simple cream shift dress under that classic navy blazer, teamed with navy shoes and bag. Smart enough for any occasion – from a school sports day to a lunch in town.

Yellow Sunny and a bit crazy, that's yellow. A good choice for swimwear, or special occasion outfits where you want to be noticed. Warmer shades of yellow are easier to wear than lemon.

Mauve Aging, sorry. If you really feel you look good in mauve, look in the mirror. Purple is even worse.

PICK STYLES THAT FLATTER YOUR FIGURE

These days, fashion is no longer dictatorial. You do not have to wear a mini-skirt, flares, an A-line dress or stilletto heels if you look silly in them. Instead, you can choose from rails and rails of different 'looks', and that's where it gets really confusing.

Stick to these rules if you want to avoid costly mistakes:

1. Forget too-short skirts if you have bad legs. Go for on-the-knee styles or wear a long skirt with a split which just shows a tantalizing glimpse of leg.

2. Wear sharp, well-cut jackets if you are big on top. Teamed with a narrow skirt, they will take inches off you.

3. Never buy anything figure-hugging in Lycra unless you are a 16-year-old 'beanpole'.

4. Always wear long sleeves if you have wobbly upper arms.

5. Wearing the same colour from head to foot makes you look taller. If you 'cut' yourself in half with a belt, you will look shorter, instantly.

6. If you have got a good bust, show it off. A hint of cleavage is always a good idea, so long as the effect is subtle. Try an uplifting bra under an almost see-through lace body with a jacket on top.

7. Always check the effect of an outfit in a long mirror so you can see if the proportions are flattering.

8. If you take a friend on a shopping spree, make sure he or she is really on your side.

9. Never be talked into buying anything you are not sure of by an over-keen shop assistant. You are bound to regret it.

10. Buy the size that fits you, even if it is a larger size than you normally take. Sizes do vary from store to store, and nothing looks worse than a too-tight outfit.

CHAPTER FIVE

YOUR 30-DAY PROGRAMME

You have read the theory behind the New You programme; now it's time for action! Set a starting date for your makeover month and stick to it. If you like, get together with a group of friends and arrange to follow the programme with them. Meet up a couple of times a week for a weigh-in and to discuss your progress. If you like, award prizes to those who shape up best. Remember, the object of the programme is not to lose masses of weight, it is to look and feel a whole lot better. You will!

Here are ten tips to help you stay the course:

1. Monitor your progress with 'before', 'during' and 'after' pictures. You have seen the spectacular photographs of our guinea-pigs, the real-life testers. Ask a friend to take a picture of you before you start, then take regular 'updates' throughout the 30 days. The final picture is bound to be special. Have it framed!

2. Read through the first seven days' diet menus, and shop for all the dry goods you need. Buy fresh produce such as salad and fruit every few days. Reserve a shelf in the fridge for your foods.

3. Check out the recipes several days in advance. Make sure you understand them (none are difficult, all are

delicious!), and have all the ingredients you need. Most of them are suitable for other members of the family, so you could need additional ingredients for making extra portions.

4. Decide when, and where, you will be doing your exercises. If you are a busy working mum, getting up half an hour earlier for an exercise session in the sitting-room could be the answer. Or, you may prefer to make time later in the day. It's up to you.

5. Read through the beauty treatments in Chapter Three. Decide which are most suitable for you, and check out those ingredients again. You may already have most of them, or simply need a quick trip to the health food shop.

6. Set yourself a goal. Earmark a special occasion, outing or trip at the end of the 30 days when it is important that you are at your best. Keep thinking about it if you are tempted to give up (although that is unlikely, I promise).

7. Tell your family what you are doing, and ask them to encourage you all the way. If your partner wants to join in, great! Several of our volunteers found that their husbands enjoyed the special programme meals and walks so much that they lost weight and shaped up as well.

8. Plot your walking route or routes. You will be walking every day so make sure you have some attractive scenery to look forward to. If you are not lucky enough to live in the country, choose a nearby park or a long, interesting street for your daily walking sessions.

9. Put all the money you save into a special pot or biscuit tin. You will be saving on petrol (all that walking!),

clothes (there's no point in buying anything for 30 days), food (you will not be eating junk or takeways), and comfort items like chocolate and alcohol. You could save enough for a new outfit in 30 days' time.

10. Keep this book with you at all times. It is your encyclopedia for the next 30 days, so you will be referring to it constantly.

N.B. The exercise levels suggested are for a person who is of average fitness. If you feel you can progress more quickly, do so. However, please do not push yourself. If you have specific problems such as a weak back or sports injury, consult your doctor, osteopath or physiotherapist.

WEEK ONE
DAY 1

WEIGH IN TODAY Weigh yourself first thing in the morning, naked, and take measurements. When you are measuring your bust or chest, remember to keep the tape-measure well up at the back. Measure waistline breathing normally (no cheating), and make sure you measure the *widest* part of your hips.

DIET

DRINKS Please drink at least 6 glasses of water or mineral water daily. I recommend Evian or one of the other still mineral waters. You may also have ½ pint (275ml) skimmed milk each day in your tea and coffee. Try to stick to decaffeinated coffee only, and limit cups to one or two a day. If you must have a diet soft drink, do so, but if possible drink more water. It is delicious with ice and lemon.

If you usually take sugar in tea or coffee, use an artificial sweetener instead. However, your taste buds will become tuned in to sugarless beverages very quickly.

ON WAKING 1 glass water with the juice of ½ lemon and artificial sweetener to taste

BREAKFAST 1oz (25g) unsweetened bran cereal (e.g. Bran Flakes), topped with sliced apple, nectarine or peach, and 2 tbsp (30ml) natural unsweetened yogurt

MID-MORNING 1 orange

LUNCH Sandwich of 2 slices wholemeal bread, 3oz (75g) tuna-in-brine, drained and mashed with lemon juice, chopped spring onion and 1 tbsp (10ml) yogurt, 1 apple

MID-AFTERNOON Selection of washed vegetables (e.g. carrot, cucumber, cauliflower, celery) with a dip made from 2 tbsp (30ml) Shape Low Fat Soft Cheese, 1 tsp (5ml) mustard, lemon juice and seasoning

SUPPER Gazpacho (*see* recipe on page 146 – make enough for tomorrow's lunch as well. Keep it chilled in the fridge), or 1 can slimmers' soup any flavour; 10oz (275g) chicken leg, roast or grilled with skin removed, Vegetable and Pasta Salad (*see* recipe on page 146), lettuce, cucumber, 1 orange. 1 cup decaffeinated coffee or tea, milk from allowance

EXERCISE PROGRAMME   (*see* page 13 onwards)

1. Complete Breath
2. Complete Posture Programme
3. Wind Down Exercise
Facial exercises (*see* page 24): Double Chin, Chubby Cheeks

WALKING Stage One

BEAUTY Beauty Bath of your choice (*see* page 28), face treatment of your choice (*see* pages 29 and 38)

SELF-IMAGE Positive Thinking Exercise

DAY 2

DIET

DRINKS As Day 1

ON WAKING 1 glass of water with the juice of 1 orange

BREAKFAST 1 slice wholemeal toast topped with grilled tomatoes (as many as you like), 2 tbsp (30ml) sweetcorn. 5oz (150g) carton natural yogurt with one chopped apple stirred in

MID-MORNING 2 plums or 1 small banana

LUNCH Gazpacho (*see* yesterday), wholemeal roll with a filling of chopped pear, lemon juice, ½ oz (15g) chopped lean ham, 1 tbsp (15ml) cottage cheese and sprigs of fresh mint

MID-AFTERNOON 1 peach, nectarine or orange

SUPPER 1 large slice of melon garnished with a slice of orange and ginger to taste, Pasta with Green Beans and Prawns (*see* recipe on page 139 – make an extra serving for tomorrow's lunch), tomato salad with sliced spring onions, parsley and 1 tbsp (15ml) Kraft Fat Free Vinaigrette Style dressing, 1 apple, 1 glass dry wine (or make two spritzers with fizzy mineral water)

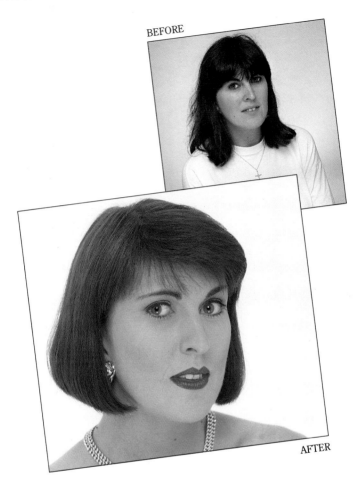

BEFORE

AFTER

Carol Barlow, 32, wanted a new look that fitted in with her busy life as a mother of three children.

Her thick dark hair was 'dragging' her face down. Joshua Galvin cut off about 8 inches, softened the fringe and ran reddish-brown highlights through the hair to give it a more textured look.

Make-up artist Jan Wright persuaded Carol to emphasize her fabulous mouth with bright red lipstick, highlighted her beautiful bone structure with blusher and used mauve and pink shadows to emphasize her eyes. Result? Stunning!

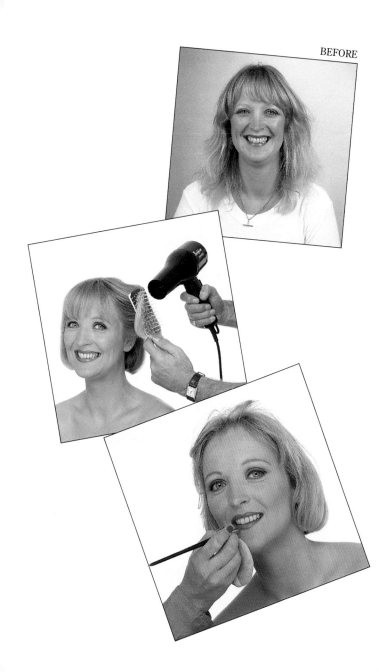

Pretty Toni Tree longed to look more stylish and had thought about having a perm so her baby-fine, naturally blonde hair was cut in two stages. The first stage would have been fine for a soft perm, but she opted for the shorter, straighter look, which is easy to keep in shape when you have children to look after.

A lip brush was used to emphasize the natural 'cupid's bow' of her mouth and Jan persuaded her to try dark brown mascara instead of the blue she used before. Brown shadows and fine brown eyeliner were perfect for her brilliant blue eyes.

To look after her sleek bobbed hair-do, Toni, 32, simply needs to wash it with a gentle shampoo and keep the ends trimmed. After rough-drying, Joshua showed her how to lift the hair from the root with a wide-toothed brush for extra volume. A very light hairspray keeps it in place.

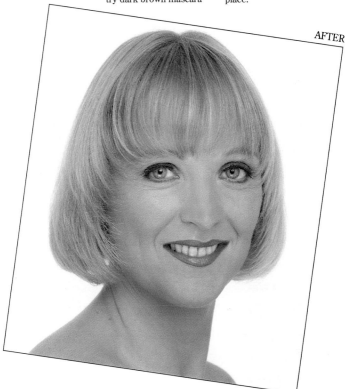

AFTER

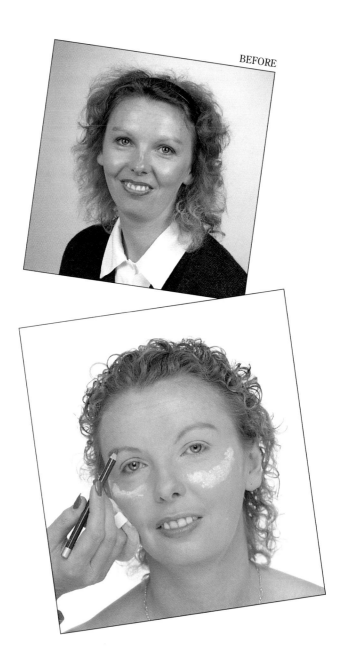

BEFORE

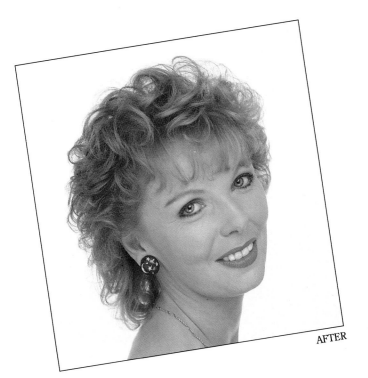

AFTER

Linda Henson, 35, had quite a few problems. Her very fine hair had the remains of an old perm in the ends, and she was desperate to have it cut and re-permed. Her brows looked sparse, and her high forehead needed disguising.

Jan 'softened' her whole face, making Linda look even younger in the process! She filled in her brows with light, feathery strokes using a soft brown eye pencil, and used grey and pink shadows on her eyes, with a little grey under her bottom lashes for extra emphasis. Loose powder on her cheek-bones stopped smudges of shadow spoiling her make-up – it was brushed away afterwards.

Her hair was permed with the ends 'blocked off' to prevent over-perming. It was cut into a softer shape, without sacrificing too much length, with a flattering fringe. She can now dry it on a round brush for the sophisticated look in our picture, or simply run her fingers through it if she's in a hurry!

Michelle Gibson, 34, has a demanding life with a two-year-old daughter to care for. She found that tying back her long, curly, naturally blonde hair was an easy option for everyday but not very flattering. She wore just a light make-up, going for a natural look, but longed to be more glamorous.

Her hair was graduated so that the fringe no longer looks 'separate' from the rest of her hair, but Joshua left it long enough to tie back if she wants to.

He also showed her how to wear her hair scrunch-dried, or roller-set with pin-set curls at the front. When the rollers were removed, each curl was clipped into place to cool, while Jan tackled Michelle's make-up. Her brows and lashes are very, very fair, so Jan advised her to have them dyed. Meanwhile, she used plenty of lash-lengthening mascara to define her eyes, plus soft grey and pink shadows.

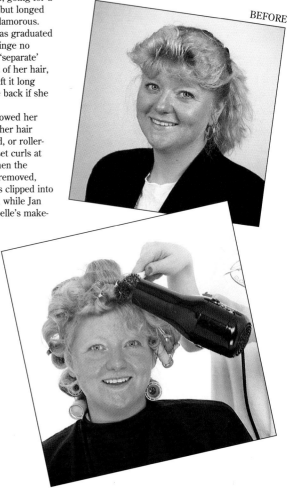

BEFORE

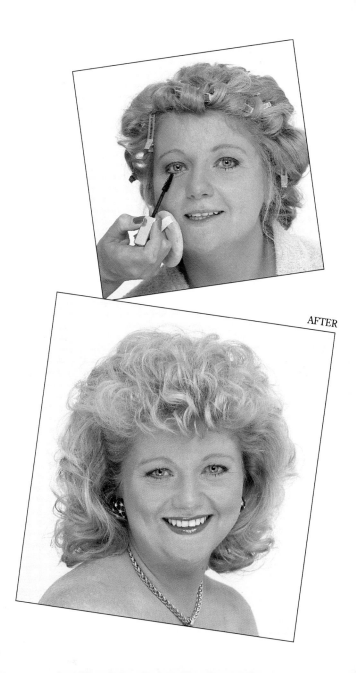

AFTER

Sue Tucker, 37, has two children aged 11 and 12 and lives in the country. She has fine, brown hair which needed shaping and re-perming. Sue was adamant that she didn't want her hair shorter, so Joshua simply added body and shape with clever cutting. He used a semi-permanent vegetable colour in a gentle reddish-blonde shade to bring out Sue's natural lights, and give a glossy look.

Her rather high colour was corrected using Rimmel's green-tinted Colour Corrector Moisturiser and Jan topped this with ivory foundation, and a natural-looking shader under her cheekbones. She advised Sue to avoid pale pink lipsticks, and go for a darker, more tawny shade instead.

All products by Rimmel
Hair by Joshua Galvin
Make-up by Jan Wright
Nickel allergy-free jewelry by Cabouchon. For catalogue and information call Caroline Marx on 071–937 4174.

BEFORE

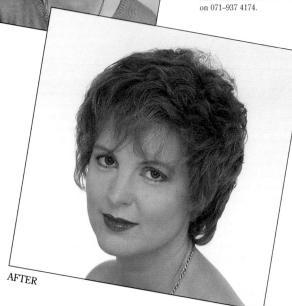

AFTER

EXERCISE PROGRAMME

1. Complete Breath
2. Complete Posture Programme
3. Stomach Muscles – Stage One
4. Bottom, Hips and Thighs – Stage One
5. Wind Down Exercise

Facial exercises: Double Chin, Chubby Cheeks

WALKING Stage One

BEAUTY Beauty Bath of your choice, face treatment of your choice, manicure (*see* page 31), massage (*see* page 34)

SELF-IMAGE Positive Thinking Programme

DAY 3

DIET

DRINKS As Day 1

ON WAKING 1 glass of water with dash of unsweetened pineapple juice and a squeeze of lemon

BREAKFAST 1 small glass unsweetened pineapple juice, 1oz (25g) bran cereal with a little skimmed milk, 1 slice wholemeal toast

MID-MORNING 1 small banana

LUNCH Cold serving of Pasta With Green Beans and Prawns (*see* yesterday's supper), sliced tomatoes, 1 small wholemeal roll

MID-AFTERNOON 1 orange

SUPPER Gammon Steak with Pineapple and Mustard Sauce (*see* recipe on page 134), 1 small jacket potato, large green salad with 1 tbsp (15ml) Kraft Fat Free

Vinaigrette Style dressing, Red Fruit Sundae (*see* recipe on page 129), or the 5oz (150g) carton strawberry-flavour diet yogurt poured over 1 chopped apple, 1 glass dry wine

EXERCISE PROGRAMME

1. Complete Breath
2. Complete Posture Programme
3. Stomach Muscles – Stage One
4. Bottom, Hips and Thighs – Stage One
5. Wind Down Exercise
Facial exercises: complete programme

WALKING Stage Two

BEAUTY Beauty Bath of your choice, hair treatment of your choice (*see* page 35)

SELF-IMAGE Positive Thinking Exercise

DAY 4

WEIGH IN TODAY Weigh yourself as on Day 1 and take measurements

DIET

DRINKS As Day 1

ON WAKING 1 glass of water with the juice of 1 orange

BREAKFAST Scrambled eggs with 2oz (50g) mushrooms poached in stock or water

MID-MORNING 1 nectarine, peach or pear

LUNCH Sandwich of 2 slices wholemeal bread with Smoked Mackerel Pâté filling (*see* recipe on page 127), 2 tomatoes

MID-AFTERNOON 1 diet yogurt, any flavour

SUPPER 6oz (175g) any white fish, grilled with lemon juice and tomatoes, 8oz (225g) jacket potato, huge mixed salad with 1 tbsp (15ml) Kraft Fat Free Vinaigrette Style Dressing

EXERCISE PROGRAMME

1. Complete Breath
2. Complete Posture Programme
3. Stomach Muscles – Stage One
4. Shoulders – Stage One
5. Bottom, Hips and Thighs – Stage One
6. Wind Down Exercise
Facial exercises: complete programme

WALKING Stage Two

BEAUTY Beauty Bath of your choice, massage, pedicure (*see* page 32)

SELF-IMAGE Positive Thinking exercises. Wear your best daytime outfit to work or to meet a friend

DAY 5

DIET

DRINKS as Day 1

ON WAKING 1 glass of water, juice of ½ lemon and artificial sweetener to taste (if you need it)

BREAKFAST 1oz (25g) bran cereal with 1 sliced apple and a little skimmed milk or apple juice, 1 slice wholemeal toast with 1 tsp (15ml) jam or honey

MID-MORNING One 5oz (150g) carton low-fat fromage frais

LUNCH Melon and Cottage Cheese Salad (*see* recipe on page 122), 1 apple

MID-AFTERNOON 2 crispbreads with 1 dsp (10ml) Shape Low-Fat Soft Cheese, sliced tomatoes

SUPPER Lamb Chops with Orange and Mint Sauce (*see* recipe on page 134), green beans, broccoli, grilled tomatoes, 1 apple, 1 glass dry wine

EXERCISE PROGRAMME

1. Complete Breath
2. Complete Posture Programme
3. Stomach Muscles – Stage One
4. Shoulders – Stage One
5. Waist – Stage One
6. Bottom, Hips and Thighs – Stage One
7. Wind Down Exercise
Facial exercises: complete programme

WALKING Stage Two

BEAUTY Beauty Bath of your choice, face treatment of your choice, foot exercises (*see* page 33), massage

SELF-IMAGE Positive Thinking Exercise

DAY 6

DIET

DRINKS As Day 1

ON WAKING 1 glass of water with juice of ½ grapefruit and sweetener to taste

BREAKFAST ½ grapefruit with a little cinnamon or ginger, 1 rasher well-grilled bacon, grilled tomatoes, 1 crispbread

MID-MORNING 1 apple

LUNCH 1 wholemeal pitta bread stuffed with lettuce, sliced tomato, 1oz (25g) lean ham, 1 tbsp (15ml) low-calorie coleslaw salad, 1 medium banana

MID-AFTERNOON 1 orange

SUPPER Stir-Fried Chicken (*see* recipe on page 136) or any Heinz Weight Watchers or Findus Lean Cuisine Chicken ready meal; a huge mixed salad with 1 tbsp (15ml) Kraft Fat Free Vinaigrette Style Dressing (or lemon juice, vinegar and herbs if you prefer), 1 small slice wholemeal bread or a small wholemeal roll, 1 glass dry white wine

EXERCISE PROGRAMME

1. Complete Breath
2. Complete Posture Programme
3. Stomach Muscle exercises – Stage Two
4. Waist – Stage Two
5. Shoulders – Stage Two
6. Bottom, Hips and Thighs – Stage Two
7. Wind Down Exercise
Facial exercises: complete programme

WALKING Stage Two

BEAUTY Beauty Bath of your choice, face treatment of your choice

SELF-IMAGEPositive Thinking – two exercises today!

DAY 7

WEIGH IN TODAY and take measurements

DIET

DRINKS As Day 1

ON WAKING 1 glass of water with the juice of 1 orange

BREAKFAST 1 slice toast topped with a small can (5oz/150g) baked beans, grilled tomatoes, 1 orange

MID-MORNING 2 plums or 1 apple

LUNCH One sandwich of 2 slices wholemeal bread, salad and 2oz (50g) Shape Low-Fat Soft Cheese, mixed with ½ oz (15g) raisins, grated carrot, chopped celery and lemon juice

MID-AFTERNOON 1 nectarine, peach or small banana

SUPPER A large serving of tomato salad with chopped chives, spring onions, basil, lemon juice, garlic and vinegar dressing; 6oz (175g) any grilled fish with Spinach Noodles (*see* recipe on page 141) or, if you hate spinach, 3oz (75g) noodles with 1 tbsp (15ml) sweetcorn and broccoli spears

EXERCISE PROGRAMME

1. Complete Breath
2. Complete Posture Programme
3. Stomach Muscles – Stage Two
4. Waist – Stage Two
5. Shoulders – Stage Two
6. Back – Stage One
7. Bottom, Hips and Thighs – Stage Three
8. Wind Down Exercise
Facial exercises: complete programme

WALKING Stage Two

BEAUTY Beauty Bath of your choice, face treatment of your choice, foot exercises, massage

SELF-IMAGE Positive Thinking Exercise. Colour Confidence Exercise: study the Colour Confidence hints on page 50, and put them into practice. For instance, create a cool image today by wearing green, or aim to look 'rich and famous' in an all-cream outfit. There is just one rule: no buying is allowed – everything you need is there in your own wardrobe.

WEEK TWO

This week you will find that the menus are slightly more generous and there is a little more alcohol. Of course, this is not essential, so do swap your wine allowance for water if you prefer.

The exercise levels are stepped up but remember *not* to overdo things. If you find that my recommended level is too difficult, drop back to Level One or Level Two. It's time to exercise the muscles that support your bust, too.

You should have a manicure and pedicure at the beginning of the week, and don't forget that relaxing massage. This is the week to start thinking about a new hairstyle and to try some make-up techniques that will make the most of your assets. After a week of facial exercises and treatments, your skin will be starting to look super!

DAY 8

WEIGH IN TODAY Weigh yourself first thing in the morning and take measurements

DIET

DRINKS As Day 1

ON WAKING 1 glass of mineral water, juice of ½ lemon, sweetener to taste

BREAKFAST 1 slice wholemeal toast, 2oz (50g) mushrooms poached in a little water, grilled tomatoes, 2 tbsp (30ml) cottage cheese (luscious on top of tomatoes with Worcestershire sauce!), 1 apple

MID-MORNING 1 peach, nectarine or small banana

LUNCH 1 mug Batchelors Slim a Soup, 1 medium wholemeal roll with salad and 1oz (25g) lean ham or chicken (no skin); 1 diet fromage frais, any flavour

MID-AFTERNOON 2 crispbreads with 2 tbsp (30ml) Shape Soft cheese, sliced tomato

SUPPER Celery, Pineapple and Walnut Salad (*see* recipe on page 143), 6oz (175g) any grilled fish or 5oz (150g) grilled pork tenderloin, grilled tomatoes, broccoli, green beans, courgettes, carrots, 1 glass dry wine

EXERCISE PROGRAMME

1. Complete Breath
2. Complete Posture Programme
3. Tummy Muscles – Stage Two
4. Waist and Midriff – Stage Two
5. Bust – Stage One
6. Back – Stage One
7. Bottom, Hips and Thighs – Stage Two
8. Wind Down Exercise
Facial exercises: complete programme

WALKING Stage Two

BEAUTY Beauty Bath of your choice, manicure

SELF-IMAGE Positive Thinking Exercise

DAY 9

DIET

DRINKS As Day 1

ON WAKING 1 glass of mineral water with juice of 1 orange

BREAKFAST 1 size 3 egg, boiled or poached, 1 slice wholemeal toast, 1 apple

MID-MORNING 1 mug Batchelors Slim a Soup, 2 sticks celery, 1 tomato

LUNCH Celery, Pineapple and Walnut Salad (*see* recipe on page 143), 1 orange

MID-AFTERNOON 1 diet yogurt or fromage frais, any flavour

SUPPER Spaghetti with Ham and Cheese Sauce (*see* recipe on page 140), huge green salad with lemon juice and vinegar dressing or 1 tbsp (15ml) Kraft Fat Free Vinaigrette Style Dressing, 1 glass dry wine

EXERCISE PROGRAMME

1. Complete Breath
2. Complete Posture Programme
3. Tummy Muscles – Stage Two
4. Waist and Midriff – Stage Two
5. Bust – Stage Two
6. Bottom, Hips and Thighs – Stage Two
7. Shoulders – Stage Two

8. Wind Down Exercise
Facial exercises: complete programme

WALKING Stage Two

BEAUTY Beauty Bath of your choice, manicure, Easy
Make-up routine

SELF-IMAGE Positive Thinking – two exercises today,
plus four Morale Boosters

DAY 10

DIET

DRINKS As Day 1

ON WAKING 1 glass of mineral water with juice or ½
grapefruit, sweetener if required

BREAKFAST ½ grapefruit, 1oz (25g) bran cereal, 1
chopped apple, 2 tbsp (30ml) apple juice

MID-MORNING 1 peach, nectarine, or small banana

LUNCH Fruity Open Sandwich (see recipe on page 125)

MID-AFTERNOON 1 mug Batchelors Slim a Soup

SUPPER Chicken and Corn Casserole (*see* recipe on
page 133), 8oz (225g) jacket potato, green beans, huge
mixed salad with lemon-juice dressing or 1 tbsp (15ml)
Kraft Fat Free Vinaigrette Style Dressing

EXERCISE PROGRAMME

1. Complete Breath
2. Complete Posture Programme
3. Tummy Muscles – Stage Two
4. Bottom, Hips and Thighs – Stage Two

5. Waist and Midriff – Stage Two
6. Bust – Stage Two
7. Shoulders – Stage Two
8. Wind Down Exercise

No Facial exercises today. Foot exercises instead!

WALKING Stage Two

BEAUTY Beauty Bath of your choice, face treatment of your choice, hair treatment

SELF-IMAGE Positive Thinking Exercise

DAY 11

WEIGH IN TODAY – and take your measurements

DIET

DRINKS As Day 1

ON WAKING 1 glass of mineral water

BREAKFAST 5oz (150g) can baked beans or spaghetti, 1 slice wholemeal toast, grilled tomatoes

MID-MORNING 1 medium glass of tomato or V8 vegetable juice, 2 crispbreads with Marmite, watercress and tomatoes

LUNCH Sandwich of 2 slices wholemeal bread, salad, 3oz (75g) tuna or salmon canned in brine, lots of lemon juice and black pepper

MID-AFTERNOON 1 diet yogurt, any flavour, 1 orange

SUPPER 5oz (150g) sirloin steak or two 3oz (75g) lamb chops, well trimmed and grilled, huge mixed salad with lemon-juice dressing or 1 tbsp (15ml) Kraft Fat Free

Vinaigrette Style Dressing, 8oz (225g) jacket potato with 2 tbsp (30ml) natural yogurt and chopped chives on top

EXERCISE PROGRAMME:

1. Complete Breath
2. Complete Posture Programme
3. Tummy Muscles – Stage Three
4. Bottom, Hips and Thighs – Stage Four
5. Bust – Stage Three
6. Wind Down Exercise

Facial exercises: complete programme

WALKING Stage Three

BEAUTY Beauty Bath of your choice, massage, treat for your feet (after all that walking, you deserve it!)

SELF-IMAGE Positive Thinking Exercise, three Morale Boosters

DAY 12

DIET

DRINKS As Day 1

ON WAKING 1 glass of mineral water with juice of 1 orange

BREAKFAST Crunchy Breakfast Special (*see* recipe on page 120 – make enough for the whole family and for tomorrow)

MID-MORNING 1 orange, apple, or pear

LUNCH 1 mug Batchelors Slim a Soup, wholemeal roll with 2oz (50g) cooked chicken (no skin) and lots of salad

MID-AFTERNOON 1 peach, nectarine or small banana

SUPPER Brown Rice and Tuna Salad (*see* recipe on page 142), large slice of melon, 1 glass dry wine

EXERCISE PROGRAMME

1. Complete Breath
2. Complete Posture Programme
3. Tummy Muscles – Stage Two
4. Bottom, Hips and Thighs – Stage Three
5. Waist and Midriff – Stage Two
6. Bust – Stage Three
7. Back – Stage One

Facial exercises: day off today!

WALKING Stage Two

BEAUTY Beauty Bath of your choice, face treatment of your choice, hair treatment of your choice

SELF-IMAGE Positive Thinking Exercise, and Colour Confidence Exercise (wear pink, if you're feeling down). Buy (or even better, borrow!) the latest fashion magazines and study the new styles. Which will suit you?

DAY 13

DIET

DRINKS As Day 1

ON WAKING 1 glass of mineral water with juice of ½ lemon, sweetener to taste

BREAKFAST Crunchy Breakfast Special (*see* recipe on page 120)

LUNCH Eastern Pitta Treat (*see* recipe on page 124)

MID-AFTERNOON 1 orange

SUPPER Tomato and Carrot Soup (*see* recipe on page 148 – make enough for tomorrow's lunch) or 1 can any slimmers' soup, 5oz (150g) lean pork tenderloin or lamb chump chop, grilled, thin gravy, courgettes, green beans, cabbage or spinach, 2 small potatoes

EXERCISE PROGRAMME

1. Complete Breath
2. Complete Posture Programme
3. Tummy Muscles – Stage Three
4. Bottom, Hips and Thighs – Stage Three
5. Waist and Midriff – Stage Two
6. Resting Back Position
7. Wind Down Exercise
Facial exercises: complete programme

WALKING Stage Two

BEAUTY Beauty Bath of your choice, face treatment of your choice, massage

SELF-IMAGE Positive Thinking exercises, two Morale Boosters. Go to the shops. Don't buy anything, but try on a few items, using the tips on page 52.

DAY 14

WEIGH IN TODAY – and take measurements

DIET

DRINKS As Day 1

ON WAKING 1 glass of mineral water with juice of ½ grapefruit, plus sweetener if required

BREAKFAST ½ grapefruit, 1 slice wholemeal toast topped with 1 rasher well-grilled back bacon, 1 tbsp (15ml) sweetcorn, grilled tomatoes

MID-MORNING 1 apple, pear or 2 plums

LUNCH Carrot and Tomato Soup (*see* yesterday's supper), 1 wholemeal roll, 1 peach or nectarine

MID-AFTERNOON 1 diet yogurt or fromage frais, any flavour

SUPPER Budapest Pork (*see* recipe on page 132) or 5oz (150g) grilled lean sirloin steak, 8oz (225g) jacket potato, huge green salad with lemon-juice dressing or 1 tbsp (15ml) Kraft Fat Free Vinaigrette Style Dressing, 1 apple, 1 glass dry wine

EXERCISE PROGRAMME

1. Complete Breath
2. Complete Posture Exercise
3. Tummy Muscles – Stage Three
4. Bottom, Hips and Thighs – Stage Three
5. Bust – Stage Three
6. Wind Down Exercise

Facial exercises: complete programme

WALKING – Stage Two

BEAUTY Beauty Bath of your choice, face treatment of your choice, foot treatment

SELF-IMAGE Positive thinking exercise, three Morale Boosters. Look at all your old junk jewelry – pick out the items that are perfect for this season's look. Put together one outfit from existing clothes and accessories in your wardrobe that is 'right on' – using ideas picked up on your shopping trip yesterday.

WEEK THREE

By now, you should be feeling some terrific benefits from your programme. Your skin and hair will be looking better, and you will notice increased energy levels. Daily tasks will seem less arduous, and you probably get tired far less easily than you did two weeks ago. Fancy, all this, and you are only half-way through!

This week is fairly strict, but you still get a little alcohol, and, of course, plenty of daily treats. This is the week to invite friends to supper, as several of the supper menus are perfect for guests. On Day 16, there is a delicious risotto dish, and on Day 20, you can feast your way through kebabs with a tangy barbecue sauce!

DAY 15

WEIGH IN TODAY – and take measurements

DIET

DRINKS As Day 1

ON WAKING juice of ½ lemon in a glass of mineral water, with sweetener to taste

BREAKFAST 1 carton natural unsweetened yogurt, or diet yogurt, any flavour, ½oz (15g) bran flakes, 1 apple, 1 tbsp raisins, served in a bowl. Half slice wholemeal toast with a little honey

MID-MORNING 1 nectarine, peach or small banana

LUNCH 1 wholemeal pitta bread stuffed with salad made from beansprouts, watercress, tomato, diced apple, 1 tbsp (15ml) natural yogurt, lemon juice, black pepper. 1 mug Batchelors Slim a Soup

MID-AFTERNOON 1 diet yogurt or fromage frais, any flavour

SUPPER Stir-Fried Vegetables with Chicken or Pork (*see* recipe on page 137), huge mixed salad with lemon-juice dressing or 1 tbsp (15ml) Kraft Fat Free Vinaigrette Style Dressing, 1 orange, 1 glass dry wine

EXERCISE PROGRAMME

1. Complete Breath
2. Complete Posture Exercise
3. Tummy Muscles – Stage Four
4. Bottom, Hips and Thighs – Stage Three
5. Waist and Midriff – Stage Two
6. Bust – Stage Three
7. Wind Down Exercise

Facial exercises: complete programme

WALKING Stage Two

BEAUTY Beauty Bath of your choice, face treatment of your choice, massage. If you need a new hairstyle, book a consultation with a good stylist. There should be no charge. Go along, armed with pictures snipped out of magazines. Then make an appointment for next week.

SELF-IMAGE Positive Thinking Exercise, two Morale Boosters. Reorganize your wardrobe, following the tips on page 47.

DAY 16

DIET

DRINKS As Day 1

ON WAKING juice of 1 orange in a glass of mineral water

BREAKFAST Spicy Banana on Toast (*see* recipe on page 122)

MID-MORNING 1 crispbread with triangle of cheese spread and 2 tomatoes

LUNCH 1 wholemeal roll with salad and 3oz (75g) sardines or pilchards, canned in tomato sauce with a few drops of lemon juice or Worcestershire sauce, chopped celery, 1 apple

MID-AFTERNOON 1 mug Batchelors Slim a Soup

SUPPER 1 large slice of melon, Prawn and Mushroom Risotto (*see* recipe on page 130), tomato and onion salad with garlic, lemon juice and seasoning

EXERCISE PROGRAMME:

1. Complete Breath
2. Complete Posture Programme
3. Tummy Muscles – Stage Four
4. Bottom, Hips and Thighs – Stage Four
5. Waist and Midriff – Stage Two
6. Bust – Stage Three
7. Shoulders – Stage Two
8. Wind Down Exercise
Facial exercises: complete programme

WALKING Stage Two

BEAUTY Beauty Bath of your choice, face treatment of your choice, pedicure, hair treatment

SELF-IMAGE: Positive Thinking Exercise, four Morale Boosters

DAY 17

DIET

DRINKS As Day 1

ON WAKING The juice of ½ grapefruit in a glass of mineral water, sweetener to taste

BREAKFAST ½ grapefruit, with ginger or cinnamon to taste, 1 slice wholemeal toast, grilled tomatoes, 1 large tbsp (15ml) cottage cheese

MID-MORNING 1 nectarine, peach or small banana

LUNCH A sandwich of 2 slices wholemeal bread with Mexican Tuna (*see* recipe on page 126) filling, or 2oz (50g) prawns with lemon juice and black pepper

MID-AFTERNOON 1 apple

SUPPER 5oz (150g) lean pork tenderloin, chicken breast or 8oz (225g) fish with Lemon Marinade (*see* recipe on page 149), 8oz (225g) jacket potato, green beans or broccoli, courgettes, cauliflower, grilled tomato, 1 glass dry wine

EXERCISE PROGRAMME

1. Complete Breath
2. Complete Posture Programme
3. Tummy Muscles – Stage Four
4. Bottom, Hips and Thighs – Stage Four
5. Waist and Midriff – Stage Two
6. Bust – Stage Three
7. Back – Stage Two
8. Wind Down Exercise
Facial exercises: none today

WALKING Stage Two

BEAUTY Beauty Bath of your choice, face treatment of your choice, massage, manicure, foot exercises

SELF-IMAGE: Positive Thinking Exercise, two Morale Boosters

DAY 18

WEIGH IN TODAY and take measurements

DIET

DRINKS As Day 1

ON WAKING The juice of 1 orange in a large glass of mineral water

BREAKFAST 1 size 3 egg, boiled or poached or 1 small can (5oz/150g) baked beans, 1 slice wholemeal toast, 1 apple

MID-MORNING 1 apple, pear or 2 plums

LUNCH 1 wholemeal roll with filling of salad and 2oz (50g) chicken or ham (no skin or fat), 1 orange

MID-AFTERNOON 1 diet yogurt or fromage frais, any flavour, a few grapes

SUPPER Tomato and Courgette Soup (*see* recipe, page 149) or Gazpacho (*see* recipe on page 146 – make enough soup for tomorrow's lunch), Bacon Steaks with Pineapple and Cheese Topping (*see* recipe on page 131), green beans, cauliflower, carrots, broccoli

EXERCISE PROGRAMME

1. Complete Breath
2. Complete Posture Programme

3. Wind Down Exercise
Facial exercises: complete programme

WALKING Stage Three today – go for it!

BEAUTY Beauty Bath of your choice, face treatment of your choice, Easy Make-up routine

SELF-IMAGE Positive Thinking Exercise, Morale Booster, Colour Confidence Exercise – wear cream or white, plus the jewelry you re-discovered last week.

DAY 19

DIET

DRINKS As Day 1

ON WAKING The juice of ½ grapefruit in a glass of mineral water, sweetener to taste

BREAKFAST 1oz (25g) bran cereal, chopped apple, 1 tbsp (15ml) sultanas, 3 tbsp (45ml) apple juice, 1 tbsp (15ml) natural, low-fat yogurt

MID-MORNING 1 nectarine, peach or small banana

LUNCH Tomato and Courgette Soup or Gazpacho (*see* yesterday's supper), or 1 can slimmer's soup, any flavour, 1 wholemeal roll, 1 diet yogurt, any flavour

MID-AFTERNOON 1 orange or 3 plums

SUPPER 1 large slice of melon, Salad Niçoise (see recipe on page 145), 3 crispbreads with 1oz (25g) low-fat hard cheese, 1 glass dry wine

EXERCISE PROGRAMME

1. Complete Breath
2. Complete Posture Programme

3. Tummy Muscles – Stage Four
4. Bottom, Hips and Thighs – Stage Four
5. Waist and Midriff – Stage Two
6. Bust – Stage Three
7. Shoulders – Stage Three
8. Wind Down Exercise
Facial exercises: complete programme

WALKING Stage Two

BEAUTY Beauty Bath of your choice, face treatment of your choice, hair treatment, massage

SELF-IMAGE Positive Thinking Exercise, three Morale Boosters

DAY 20

DIET

DRINKS As Day 1

ON WAKING juice of ½ grapefruit in mineral water, sweetener to taste

BREAKFAST ½ grapefruit, 1 slice wholemeal toast with 1 tsp jam or marmalade, diet yogurt, any flavour

LUNCH A sandwich of 2 slices wholemeal bread, salad 1oz (25g) low-fat hard cheese, grated and mixed with 1 dsp low-calorie mayonnaise, 1 tomato, 1 apple

MID-AFTERNOON Washed, sliced vegetables with dip made from 1 tbsp (15ml) Shape Soft Cheese, 1 tbsp (15ml) natural, unsweetened yogurt, with a dash of tomato ketchup, Tabasco and lemon juice

SUPPER Lamb or Pork Kebabs with Barbecue Sauce (*see* recipe on page 135), huge mixed salad with lemon-juice dressing or 1 tbsp (15ml) Kraft Fat Free Vinaigrette Style Dressing.

EXERCISE PROGRAMME

1. Complete Breath
2. Complete Posture Programme
3. Tummy Muscles – Stage Four
4. Bottom, Hips and Thighs – Stage Four
5. Waist and Midriff – Stage Two
6. Bust – Stage Three
7. Wind Down Exercise

Facial exercises: none today

WALKING Stage Two

BEAUTY Beauty Bath of your choice, Easy Make-up routine, pedicure, massage, foot exercises

SELF IMAGE: Positive Thinking Exercise, three Morale Boosters

DAY 21

WEIGH IN TODAY – and take measurements

DIET

DRINKS As Day 1

ON WAKING juice of 1 orange in 1 glass of mineral water

BREAKFAST Fruity Breakfast Roll (*see* recipe on page 121)

MID-MORNING 1 orange, pear or small banana

LUNCH 1 large slice of melon, 10oz (275g) chicken piece, grilled or roast, no skin, huge mixed salad with Spicy Tomato Juice Dressing (*see* recipe on page 127)

MID-AFTERNOON 1 apple, a few grapes

SUPPER ½ grapefruit, 8oz (225g) any grilled white fish, 8oz (225g) jacket potato, courgettes, green beans or cauliflower, Orange and Watercress Salad (*see* recipe on page 145), a few grapes, 1 glass dry wine

EXERCISE PROGRAMME

1. Complete Breath
2. Complete Posture Exercise
3. Tummy Muscles – Stage Four
4. Bottom, Hips and Thighs – Stage Four
5. Bust – Stage Three
6. Back – Stage Two
7. Wind Down Exercise
Facial exercises: complete programme

WALKING Stage Two

BEAUTY Beauty Bath of your choice, face treatment of your choice, massage

SELF-IMAGE Two Positive Thinking exercises, four Morale Boosters

WEEK FOUR

The diet, this week, is a little tougher to start with, but don't worry because it does get easier. Do not forget to drink plenty of water every day. If you have booked a hair appointment this week, make sure you have allowed plenty of time. There is nothing worse than sitting watching the clock tick away while you are having a perm or colour treatment, knowing that you have to rush back to work. This is also the week to buy yourself something new to wear but remember that it doesn't have to be expensive. A bright jacket, sweater or skirt could liven up existing outfits in your wardrobe.

The final two days are very easy indeed with a generous menu and a slightly less strenuous exercise programme. However, if you have more weight to lose, I do suggest that you do the whole programme once again, adjusting the exercise levels according to your ability.

Whether you are in perfect shape or not, do plan a special outing for Day 31, when you can show off your new look.

(For those who have reached their 'happy' weight and feel very satisfied with the results of the programme, there is a Maintenance Plan on page 110.)

DAY 22

WEIGH IN TODAY – and take measurements

DIET

DRINKS As Day 1

ON WAKING The juice of ½ lemon in 1 glass mineral water, sweetener to taste

BREAKFAST 1oz (25g) bran flakes, medium banana, a little skimmed milk

MID-MORNING 1 orange

LUNCH A sandwich of 2 slices wholemeal bread, salad and 2oz (50g) chicken or ham (no skin or fat), 1 apple

MID-AFTERNOON 1 diet yogurt or fromage frais, any flavour, 1 small banana

SUPPER Bangers (sausages) with Rice (*see* recipe on page 131), cauliflower, cabbage, green beans, courgettes, carrots

EXERCISE PROGRAMME

1. Complete Breath
2. Complete Posture Exercise
3. Tummy Muscles – Stage Five
4. Bottom, Hips and Thighs – Stage Four
5. Waist and Midriff – Stage Two
6. Bust – Stage Three
7. Shoulders – Stage Three
8. Wind Down Exercise

Facial exercises: complete programme

WALKING Stage Three

BEAUTY Beauty Bath of your choice, face treatment of your choice, pedicure, massage

SELF-IMAGE Positive Thinking Exercise, three Morale Boosters

DAY 23

DIET

DRINKS As Day 1

ON WAKING The juice of 1 orange in mineral water

BREAKFAST 1 size 3 egg, poached on 1 slice wholemeal toast, grilled tomatoes

MID-MORNING 1 nectarine, peach or small banana

LUNCH Pasta Waldorf Salad (*see* recipe on page 123), 1 small wholemeal roll

MID AFTERNOON 1 diet yogurt, any flavour

SUPPER 10oz (275g) chicken piece (no skin), grilled or roast, Courgettes with Lime and Cumin (*see* recipe on page 150), mixed salad with lemon-juice dressing or 1 tbsp (15ml) Kraft Fat Free Vinaigrette Style Dressing

EXERCISE PROGRAMME

1. Complete Breath
2. Complete Posture Exercise
3. Tummy Muscles – Stage Five
4. Bottom, Hips and Thighs – Stage Five
5. Waist and Midriff – Stage Two
6. Bust – Stage Three
7. Wind Down Exercise

Facial exercises: full programme

WALKING Stage Two

BEAUTY Beauty Bath of your choice, face treatment of your choice, hair treatment, pedicure, foot exercises – full programme

SELF-IMAGE Two Positive Thinking exercises, two Morale Boosters, shopping expedition – spend a little on yourself!

DAY 24

DIET

DRINKS As Day 1

ON WAKING The juice of ½ grapefruit in mineral water, sweetener to taste.

BREAKFAST ½ grapefruit, 1 slice wholemeal toast topped with small can (5oz/150g) baked beans, grilled tomatoes, watercress

MID MORNING 1 mug Batchelors Slim a Soup, 2 crispbreads

LUNCH Wholemeal pitta, split and filled with lettuce, cucumber and Salmon Pâté (*see* recipe on page 127 – make enough for tomorrow's supper), 1 apple

MID-AFTERNOON 1 nectarine, peach or small banana

SUPPER Cod in a Parcel (*see* recipe on page 129), 7oz (200g) jacket potato, green beans or courgettes, grilled tomatoes, 2 tbsp (30ml) sweetcorn, huge mixed salad with lemon-juice dressing or 1 tbsp (15ml) Kraft Fat Free Vinaigrette Style Dressing

EXERCISE PROGRAMME

1. Complete Breath
2. Complete Posture Exercise
3. Tummy Muscles – Stage Five
4. Bottom, Hips and Thighs – Stage Five
5. Waist and Midriff – Stage Two
6. Back – Stage Two
Facial exercises: forget them today!

WALKING Stage Three

BEAUTY Beauty Bath of your choice, face treatment of your choice, Easy Make-up routine

SELF IMAGE Positive Thinking exercise, two Morale Boosters. You should have lunch out with a friend today, and wear red!

DAY 25

WEIGH IN TODAY – and take measurements

DIET

DRINKS As Day 1

ON WAKING The juice of ½ lemon in mineral water with sweetener to taste

BREAKFAST 1 slice wholemeal toast with 1 tsp (5ml) honey or marmalade, 1 apple

MID-MORNING 1 diet yogurt or fromage frais, any flavour

LUNCH Cheesy Fish Grill (*see* recipe on page 124) or wholemeal roll with salad and 3oz (75g) tuna-in-brine, plus plenty of lemon juice and black pepper, 1 orange

MID-AFTERNOON 2 crispbreads with Marmite, sliced tomatoes and watercress

SUPPER Salmon Pâté (*see* yesterday's lunch) with 1 slice toast, 3oz (75g) any pasta with Herby Tomato Sauce (*see* recipe on page 125), huge green salad with lemon-juice dressing or 1 tbsp (15ml) Kraft Fat Free Vinaigrette Style Dressing

EXERCISE PROGRAMME

1. Complete Breath
2. Complete Posture Programme
3. Tummy Muscles – Stage Five
4. Bottom, Hips and Thighs – Stage Five
5. Waist and Midriff – Stage Two
6. Wind Down Exercise

Facial exercises: complete programme

BEAUTY Beauty Bath of your choice, Easy Make-up routine, professional hair cut or perm today

SELF-IMAGE Positive Thinking Exercise, one Morale Booster. Spend a long time in front of a mirror ... you are looking good!

DAY 26

DIET

DRINKS As Day 1

ON WAKING The juice of 1 orange in mineral water

BREAKFAST Gypsy Toast (*see* recipe on page 121), or 2 rashers well-grilled streaky bacon with grilled tomatoes

MID-MORNING 1 nectarine, peach or small banana

LUNCH 10 oz (275g) jacket potato or 3 oz (75g) cooked pasta with one serving Herby Tomato Sauce (*see* recipe on page 125) and 1 oz (25g) grated low-fat hard cheese plus a huge mixed salad with lemon-juice dressing or 1 tbsp (15ml) Kraft Fat Free Vinaigrette Style Dressing. OR A sandwich of 2 slices wholemeal bread spread thinly with Herby Tomato Sauce (*see* above), 2 tbsp cottage cheese, cucumber, lettuce, watercress

MID-AFTERNOON 1 apple

SUPPER Sweet and Sour Pork Fillet (*see* recipe on page 138), cauliflower, carrots, cabbage, large green salad with lemon-juice dressing

EXERCISE PROGRAMME

1. Complete Breath
2. Complete Posture Programme
3. Tummy Muscles – Stage Five
4. Bottom, Hips and Thighs – Stage Five
5. Waist and Midriff – Stage Two
6. Wind Down Exercise
Facial exercises: rest day today!

WALKING Back to Stage Two, or stick with Stage Three if it was easy yesterday

BEAUTY Beauty Bath of your choice, massage, Easy Make-up routine

SELF-IMAGE   Positive Thinking Exercise. Check through all accessories in your wardrobe. Take down-at-heel shoes to be repaired, throw out those beyond repair. Clean bags and shoes.

DAY 27

DIET

DRINKS As Day 1

ON WAKING The juice of ½ lemon in mineral water, with artificial sweetener to taste

BREAKFAST   ½ medium melon, deseeded, flesh chopped and mixed with 1 tbsp (15ml) bran flakes, and 1 chopped apple. Pile back in shell and pour over a diet yogurt, any flavour

MID-MORNING   2 crispbreads spread with Marmite, sliced tomatoes, watercress

LUNCH 1 wholemeal roll with lettuce, watercress and Prawn Cocktail filling (*see* recipe on page 126), 1 mug Batchelors Slim a Soup, any flavour

MID-AFTERNOON 1 nectarine, peach or small banana

SUPPER Leek and Potato Soup (*see* recipe on page 147 – make enough for tomorrow's lunch), or 1 can any slimmer's soup, served chilled or hot, 5 oz (150g) well-grilled lean lamb chop or rump steak, grilled tomatoes, huge mixed salad with lemon-juice dressing or 1 tbsp (15ml) Kraft Fat Free Vinaigrette Style Dressing

EXERCISE PROGRAMME

Take a break from your normal routine, and go swimming instead. Swim up and down for at least 20 minutes, non-stop, at your own pace.
Facial exercises: complete programme

WALKING Stage Two

BEAUTY Beauty Bath of your choice, massage, foot treatment, Easy Make-up routine

SELF-IMAGE Positive Thinking Exercise, book up your treat for Day 31! It could be an outing to a concert, a theatre trip, a night out at a club.

DAY 28

WEIGH IN TODAY – and take measurements

DIET

DRINKS As Day 1

ON WAKING The juice of ½ grapefruit in mineral water, sweetener to taste

BREAKFAST ½ grapefruit, with cinnamon or ginger to taste, 1 oz (25g) bran cereal, a little skimmed milk

MID-MORNING 1 carton diet yogurt, any flavour

LUNCH Leek and Potato Soup (*See* yesterday's supper), 2 crispbreads, 1 oz (25g) hard cheese, 1 tomato, 1 apple

MID-AFTERNOON 1 nectarine, peach or small banana

SUPPER Chicken Salad Supreme (*see* recipe on page 143), a large helping of frozen raspberries topped with 1 tbsp (15ml) fromage frais, 1 glass dry wine

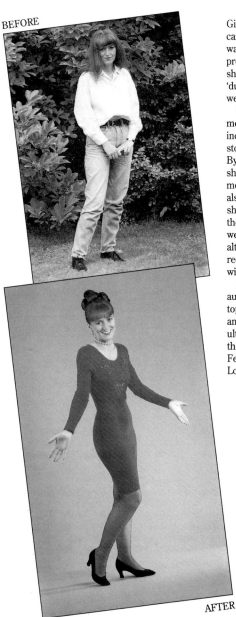

BEFORE

AFTER

Gina Rea, 33, is a busy career girl who simply wanted to tone up on our programme. She felt that she was getting rather 'dumpy', and her jeans were tight!

She's 5ft 4in tall and measured 34–25–37 inches and weighed 9½ stone when she started. By the end of the 30 days she weighed 8st 12lb and measured 34–24–35. She also felt great! Amazingly, she managed to stick to the programme during a week's holiday in Italy, although this is not recommended for anyone without terrific willpower!

Her thick, natural auburn hair was piled on top for a different look, and she can now wear ultra-clingy dresses like this party number from Fenwicks of Bond Street, London.

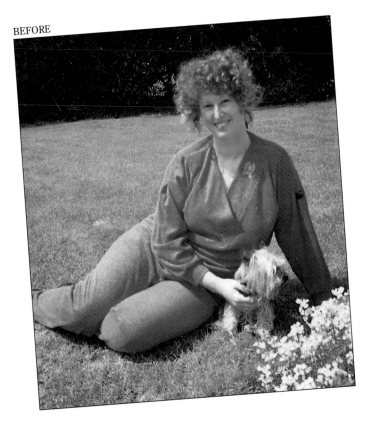

Cathy Whiting, 37, weighed in at 13st 4lb and measured 43–34½–46 inches when she started the programme. She is tall (5ft 7in) and has a large frame, but she felt that she needed to lose quite a bit of weight and change her look. Pretty Cathy is married and works as a doctor's receptionist.

The programme proved to Cathy that the right clothes can help you look slimmer even if you don't lose much weight (she actually shed 9lb, and lost 2 inches off her bust and 3 inches off her hips). The long-line red jacket, trim white skirt and striped shirt from Fenwicks, gave her a leaner, more flattering line and showed off her great legs!

She says: 'I will throw away my baggy tracksuits and wear skirts from now on!'

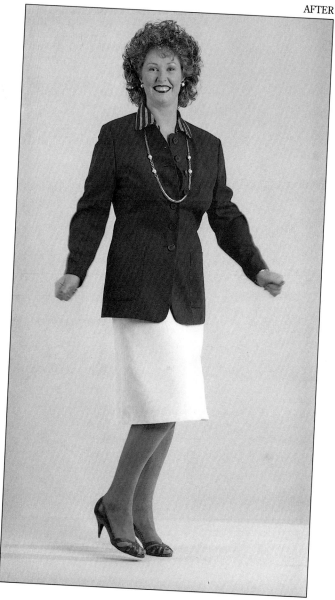

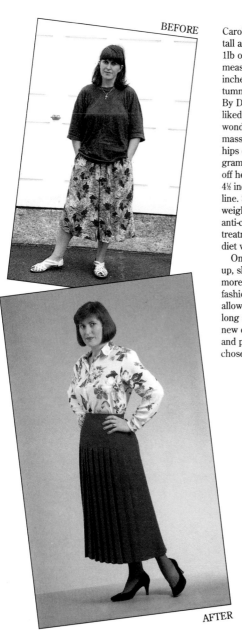

BEFORE

AFTER

Carol Barlow is 5ft 5½in tall and she weighed 12st 1lb on Day 1. She measured 39½–32–47 inches. She hated her tummy, bottom and legs. By Day 30, she quite liked all three! No wonder. Carol, 32, lost a massive *7 inches* off her hips during the programme, plus 3 inches off her bust and 4½ inches off her waistline. She also lost 10lb in weight. She says: 'The anti-cellulite beauty treatment, exercises and diet worked wonders.'

Once she had shaped up, she opted for a much more figure-hugging fashion style, which still allowed her to wear the long skirts she loves. Her new outfit, a well-cut shirt and pleated skirt, was chosen from C & A.

When she started the 30 Day Programme, Toni Tree, 32, was fed up with wearing the young mums' 'uniform' of leggings and baggy top. She weighed 11st 10½lb, about 3 stone too much for her 5ft 3in frame, and measured 38–32–44 inches. She also had cellulite around her hips and bottom.

Toni was determined to succeed, so she used a pair of tight jeans to measure her progress. She lost 16½lb and shrank to 35–27½–40½. Her now-baggy jeans prove how effective the plan was.

She says: 'This is the kind of picture that is often faked for diet pill advertisements. In my case, it's absolutely genuine. I am keeping the jeans, as an awful reminder of just how large I was!'

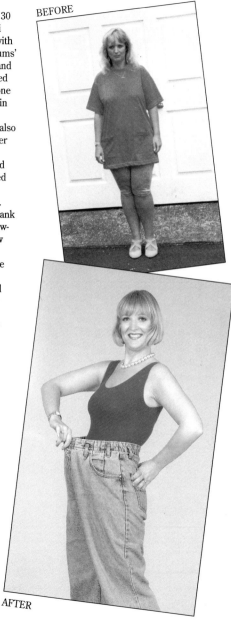

AFTER

Linda Henson was another 'leggings and sloppy top' girl with a very good figure which had simply thickened up a little since the births of her two children. She trimmed down from 10st 4lb, 35–29½–40½ inches to 9st 8lb, 34–26–37, perfect for her height, 5ft 7in.

Linda, 35, says: 'I never dared wear anything too sophisticated before in case I looked silly. But I really do feel good in this gorgeous beige suit. I have thrown away my leggings – forever!' Her suit is from the London fashion boutique, Moa.

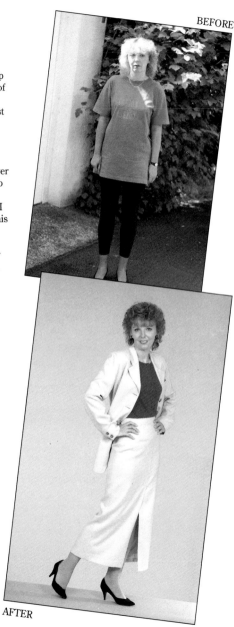

BEFORE

AFTER

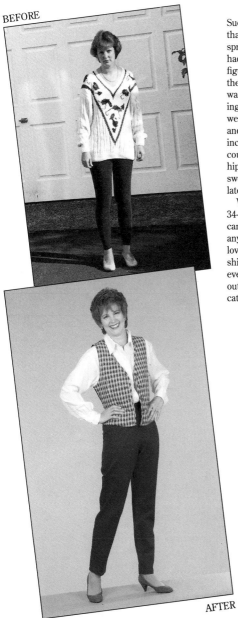

BEFORE

Sue Tucker was worried that her hips were spreading. In fact, she had a basically good figure when she started the programme, but it was in danger of becoming pear-shaped. She weighed exactly 10st and measured 34–29–39 inches. At 5ft 7in, she could easily disguise her hips with long-line sweaters. Thirty days later, she didn't have to!

With her new, 9st 5lb, 34–26–36½ figure, Sue can, and does, wear anything with style. She loves the look of trousers, shirt and waistcoat for everyday, and chose this outfit from a Freemans catalogue.

AFTER

Joy Hawkins works for a television company and spends her days researching and writing. Joy, who's 48 and has a 19-year-old daughter, has to attend a lot of programme-planning meetings and felt that her image was a bit too 'homely'. Although she didn't have much weight to lose, the programme gave her the push she needed to revamp her image.

She trimmed down from 9st 2lb, 36–28–36 inches to 8st 12lb, and shaped up beautifully on the exercise and walking plans. The beauty routines forced her to spend more time on herself. Her expensive-looking scarlet jacket and black skirt came from C & A, which proves that you don't have to spend a lot to look high-powered.

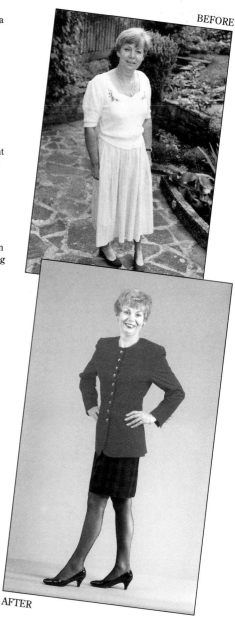

BEFORE

AFTER

EXERCISE PROGRAMME

1. Complete Breath
2. Complete Posture Exercise
3. Tummy Muscles – Stage Five
4. Bottom, Hips and Thighs – Stage Five
5. Waist and Midriff – Stage Two
6. Bust – Stage Two
7. Wind Down Exercise

Facial exercises: complete programme

WALKING Stage Three

BEAUTY Beauty Bath of your choice, face treatment of your choice

SELF-IMAGE Positive thinking exercise, four Morale Boosters

FINAL TWO DAYS

DAY 29

DIET

DRINKS As Day 1

ON WAKING The juice of ½ lemon in mineral water, sweetener to taste

BREAKFAST Nutty Orange Sunshine Breakfast (*see* recipe on page 121), 1 slice wholemeal toast with 1tsp jam or marmalade.

MID-MORNING 1 apple

LUNCH A sandwich of 2 slices wholemeal bread, 3oz (75g) tuna in brine with lemon juice, 1 tomato

MID-AFTERNOON 1 diet yogurt or fromage frais, any flavour

SUPPER 10oz (275g) grilled chicken piece, no skin or fat, Mushroom and Beansprout Salad (*see* recipe on page 144), 1 scoop vanilla icecream with sliced banana, nectarine or peach

EXERCISE PROGRAMME

Full programme: at the level you feel comfortable with. Facial exercises: full programme

WALKING Stage Three

BEAUTY Beauty Bath of your choice, Easy Make-up routine, pedicure

SELF-IMAGE Positive Thinking Exercise

DAY 30

FINAL WEIGH-IN – and take measurements

DIET

DRINKS As Day 1

ON WAKING The juice of 1 orange in mineral water

BREAKFAST 1 egg, boiled or poached, 1 slice wholemeal toast, 1 medium glass unsweetened orange or grapefruit juice

MID-MORNING 1 apple, pear or small banana

LUNCH 2 Ryvita Crispbreads, 1 serving Spinach and Soft Cheese Pâté (*see* recipe on page 128), 1 diet yogurt or fromage frais, any flavour

MID-AFTERNOON A selection of washed, sliced vegetables with dip made from 2 tbsp (30ml) natural yogurt, 1 tsp (5ml) each mustard, lemon juice and mixed herbs

SUPPER Pasta with Fresh Tomato Sauce (*see* recipe on page 140), huge mixed salad with lemon-juice dressing or 1 tbsp (15ml) Kraft Fat Free Vinaigrette Style Dressing, 1 apple, pear or small banana, 1 glass dry wine

EXERCISE PROGRAMME

As Day 29
Skip facial exercises!

WALKING Stage Two

BEAUTY Beauty Bath of your choice, face treatment of your choice, massage, Easy Make-up routine

SELF-IMAGE Look in the mirror. Feel great? You should!

CHAPTER SIX

OUR TESTERS' DIARIES

I asked each of the volunteers who tested the 30-Day programme to keep a daily diary. In it, each guinea-pig noted down her daily thoughts, reaction to the diet, how she felt, her progress on the various exercise routines, walking and the psychological side of the programme. If you do the same, you will find you'll be able to stay the course much more successfully, and you will also find that some of your diary notes are extremely revealing. As you progress, it will be fun to check back and see just how you felt right at the beginning.

Here are some extracts from the diaries of five of our volunteers, plus their 'before' and 'after' records.

Name: **Toni Tree**
Age: **32** *Height*: **5ft 3in**
Starting weight: **11st 10½lb**
Weight after 30 days: **10st 8lb**
Total weight loss: **16½lb**
Starting measurements: **38–32–44 inches**
Measurements after 30 days: **35–27½–40½ inches**

DAY 1 Great! A new day, a new start, and the start of a new, new me. I'm all fired up and ready to go. Here goes the first glass of water – only another 239!

I'm shopping for seven days' meals today. There's so much fruit and vegetables that my trolley will be over-flowing.

Gosh, it's 2.15 p.m., and I haven't cheated yet. I don't even feel hungry. Water, water everywhere, and every drop I have to drink . . . phew!

Later: I loved the Vegetable and Pasta Salad.

DAY 5 Got on the scales today. I've lost 5lbs. I can't believe it. Surely this can't keep on happening throughout the 30 days? I feel really good, but didn't like the lunch very much. Enjoyed dinner, though . . . I just love lamb chops!

DAY 8 What a delicious breakfast. I hope the second week will be as good as the first. Enjoyed lunch, too. Didn't have my afternoon snack, as I didn't feel hungry . . . will have it later on.

Went to see my brother and sister-in-law and, hor-rors, they had a takeaway pizza. I had just a slice of melon and some strawberries, and had my fish at home. Got back too late for my Beauty Bath, though. I'll have an extra long wallow tomorrow.

DAY 11 Loved the spaghetti on toast. My chin is cov-ered in spots. My skin hasn't been this bad since my teens, so maybe things are being flushed out. Hope this part of the 'makeover' is short-lived!

Fish again, good job I like it. Didn't feel very hungry tonight, but very tired after a long, long walk. Hope the scales have moved again tomorrow.

DAY 12 Oh boy, what a scrummy brekki! I could eat this every day. Looks as if the scales have moved. Yippee, I'm nearer to that magical 10 stone.

Lunch tasted better than I thought it was going to. I seem to have a spring in my step, and the spots are clearing. Hope I don't end up the same shape as a nectarine, I am eating so many of them!

DAY 14 Grumpy today. Feel as though I have spread, although I know I haven't. It must be pre-menstrual bloating. What will I do when I get the dreaded sugar cravings?

Lunch was fine and I loved the Budapest Pork recipe, but the family moaned about it. I had my bath and banana, yogurt, and honey face mask. I should have eaten it instead . . . what a mess! Skin looked okay afterwards, though.

DAY 15 Feel in a better mood today, but still don't feel slim. Really enjoyed supper. My husband helped chop and cook the Stir-Fried Vegetables with Chicken.

I went to a step class and did all my exercises. I feel really tired tonight.

DAY 17 Booked next year's holiday today. I can't wait to show off my new figure. All the bloating has disappeared and I have almost 'cracked' the 11 stone barrier. Wow!

I am really into this now, and I don't even want naughty things. I burned off a few extra calories at a fun fair with the children. Had bags of energy.

DAY 19 I wore my super leather suit today, which I haven't been able to get into for ages. Felt really good. Went to friends for dinner, but rang up first to arrange my own meal. What a cheek! But, I felt really good tucking into my meal while everyone else ate a huge pork roast.

People are starting to notice and comment on how I look. I can stand any amount of flattery. Lovely!

DAY 20 Got on the scales first thing this morning . . .

yes, it's 11 stone. In a couple of days I will be 10 stone something. Great! I feel really good today. I have started taking Alexandra with me on her bike so I have to walk briskly to keep up with her.

I was glad that I had soup instead for lunch as it was a cold day. I did all the exercises and the facial ones must be doing something . . . my muscles really ache!

DAY 21 The breakfast was very filling. I did my exercise tape, then took the children swimming and shopping. I feel so much better eating properly that I don't think I'll ever go back to my old eating habits.

On my walk today, I bumped into someone I haven't seen for quite a while and she didn't recognize me. I felt wonderful.

DAY 22 I got my first wolf whistle for six years! I was so shocked that I turned around to see if it was for someone else, then realized that I was alone, so it must have been for me.

I was wearing a knee-length skirt and body suit as part of my positive-thinking programme – maybe the outfit had something to do with the whistle!

The incident gave me the courage to book a consultation with a hairdresser. I've been longing to have my hair cut in a shorter, more modern style for ages. I really enjoyed tonight's Bangers and Rice – I didn't think I would be eating sausages again!

DAY 24 I swam 34 lengths (½ mile) and walked nearly two miles today. What a mover! Went to a party, and enjoyed dressing up. I wore a little black number that had been pushed to the back of the wardrobe.

Guess what I found when I stripped off to get changed? Yes, hip bones! After six years, they are actually still there. My husband is really thrilled, and so am I.

DAY 26 Went to the hairdresser's today, and had my cut. I love it! The style is perfect for my fine blonde hair. Was a bit worried what the children and my husband would think. I needn't have worried, they loved it too.

Practised the Easy Make-Up again. I have now got it down to a fine art, and can get myself together in about half an hour, even with the new hair-do!

DAY 29 Took the children swimming and felt so much better in my swimsuit. I did loads of entertaining today – aunts, uncles, sister-in-law and children. I actually slipped up and had two biscuits, but found that I could actually STOP at two. Before starting the programme, I would have eaten the whole packet.

DAY 30 What a great day. It buzzed for me. I weighed in and found I was 10 stone 8lb. I was just speechless, which is very rare indeed.

I loved all my exercises today, and my walk was invigorating. I really enjoyed the Pasta with Fresh Tomato Sauce tonight. The question is: can I repeat the programme for another month? The answer just *has* to be 'yes'.

Toni did repeat the programme and now weighs under 10 stone. She keeps in trim with regular exercise and walking and looks absolutely terrific.

Name: **Linda Henson**
Age: **35** *Height*: **5ft 7in**
Starting weight: **10st 4lb**
Weight after 30 days: **9st 8lb**
Total weight loss: **10lb**
Starting measurements: **35–29½–40½ inches**
Measurements after 30 days: **34–26–37 inches**

DAY 1 I've been looking forward to this day. I was a bit worried that I wouldn't get out of bed without my usual pot of tea, but I found the water and lemon refreshing. We went out for the day, so I took my packed lunch with me. I walked to the shops and back which took an hour. My legs felt very wobbly and I was tired. I must be very unfit!

After supper, I slipped into a lovely scented bath and did some positive thinking on the new me. Only another 29 days to go . . .

DAY 2 Woke up with a headache, but it went after breakfast. I had to get Gary, my husband, to read out the exercises while I did them. I hit Gary and a lampshade once swinging my arms and legs about. I like these beauty baths: I find them relaxing and I dream of the new me while I soak.

DAY 5 Did my exercises alone this morning, as I have now got the hang of them. Only the cat watched! I do them in front of the mirror wearing only underwear so I can see my posture and ribs stretching with the Complete Breath exercise.

I do feel slimmer and very pleased with myself. Loved the lunch today. I went out to a birthday barbecue but managed to stick to the supper, almost! I am very proud of myself.

DAY 7 Walked to Oxted and back today, and enjoyed it. I think I'll leave the car at home more often. I feel very pleased with the diet and haven't craved any 'forbidden' foods. My skin is much clearer. Decided to remove my baggy top and leggings 'uniform' today and wear a skirt. Yes, I have got legs, and a waist.

I have now lost 4 lb.

DAY 9 Feel great. I loved the Spaghetti with Ham and Cheese Sauce. I would happily give this to guests. I tried the oily skin mask with melon, yogurt and egg white, but I didn't whisk it enough, and it kept sliding off my face. So, I then tried the porridge oats as washing grains. This was great. I have always bought cleansing grains before, which can be too rough. Porridge is brilliant and a whole lot cheaper.

Tried on a little black velvet number bought a year ago and never worn. It looks good and if I can shape up my hips and thighs, it will look even better!

DAY 12 Went to see Mum and Dad today. They haven't seen me for a week and couldn't believe the change in me. I went shopping in Sutton and tried on lots of clothes that wouldn't have suited me before. In the changing room, I caught sight of my rear view, and was pleased, for once.

I did 15 lengths in the swimming pool, ten short of my target but the wave machine was on, so it was more strenuous.

DAY 16 We walked from Tandridge to Godstone which is a 5-mile round trip. Felt great and not tired at all. We didn't get back until 3 p.m., and I hadn't had lunch, but I didn't feel hungry – had it anyway. I must stick to the rules!

The banana on toast this morning must have been

really filling. Or perhaps the water is making me feel full? I don't crave my old favourites, cheese, chips and icecream. I certainly won't be going back to my old eating habits when the 30 days are over.

DAY 18 I've noticed my thighs and upper arms are toning up beautifully, so the exercise is obviously doing me good. The walks are part of my life now, and I hardly ever take the car. I weighed in today, and haven't lost anything but the inches are coming off. I am wearing clothes that used to be too tight just three weeks ago. It's like having a whole new wardrobe.

DAY 20 A crisis day ... a day for breaking diets and eating everything in sight. I went to work and was told that I can't go back because of a drop in the numbers of children at the nursery. I feel very low, but I'm trying to think positively. Perhaps the new me is ready for a change? I could easily have broken my diet today, but it's now 10 p.m. and I haven't yet. Later: had a medicinal glass of wine, but the sparkle is back, and I know I've done something positive today, even though the news was negative.

DAY 22 Went on an extra long walk today, just to buy a pint of milk. Tried the porridge facial scrub again. It's great. Went out to my friend Sue's house for dinner. She is following the programme too, so she made a meal from it. The men just had extra rice with it. We are all very impressed with the recipes.

DAY 25 I went and had my new hair-do today. At last, I've found a style that really looks good on me. The soft fringe does wonders for my face shape, disguising my high forehead. Stuck to the diet brilliantly, taking my lunch along to the hairdresser's with me.

DAY 29 Decided I needed some new clothes as even the old ones that were too tight are now too big. I'll have to save up. I bought some make-up and practised making up my eyes to make them look bigger. I know I'll have to practise but this part is fun. I now seem to have time to look after me. Perhaps I always had the time before but just didn't bother to use it.

DAY 30 Weighed in and I've lost 10lb. I feel marvellous, too. Full of energy and on top of the world. This programme has really changed my life. I am happy with my weight, now, for the first time in years. I'll go on the Maintenance Plan, and try to maintain my weight and shape forever. Hope I can!

Linda has kept her weight down to 9 stone 8lb since finishing the 30-day programme and she has a new job.

Name **Carol Barlow**
Age: **32** *Height:* **5ft 5½ in**
Starting weight: **12st 1lb**
Weight after 30 days: **11st 5lb**
Total weight loss: **10lb**
Starting measurements: **39½–32–47 inches**
Measurements after 30 days: **36½–27½–40 inches**

DAY 1 Woke up with a headache this morning and thought 'What a great start'. Luckily, it soon went away and I am now feeling really positive that I can do this. My three children helped with the exercises and had a great time. I had forgotten how nice raw vegetables are. Didn't like the Gazpacho very much but loved the Vegetable and Pasta Salad.

DAY 4 It's funny waking up and *not* thinking of food straight away. I'm enjoying the walking, but have 'upped' my exercise levels slightly as they were too easy before. I really want to lose inches off my hips. The perfumed bath was relaxing and luxurious. Imagined I was in a health spa!

DAY 5 It was my son's eleventh birthday today and we took him to a burger restaurant where I would normally have 'pigged out'. But not today. Instead, I did some positive thinking and realized that it wasn't worth breaking the diet!

DAY 7 We started our holiday at a camp by the sea today, and I am worried about sticking to the diet. We're self-catering though, so I should be fine. There's no bath where we are staying, only a shower, so I pointed the shower at my wobbly bits and scrubbed really hard instead of doing my usually anti-cellulite treatment. My legs ache from swimming yesterday.

DAY 13 Last day of our holiday and I did my exercises brilliantly. Have come to the conclusion that it is very difficult to stick to a diet on holiday, but not impossible. I can't wait to see what the scales say. It will be great to be home and able to indulge in some of the beauty baths again.

DAY 14 I am absolutely thrilled at the way the inches are coming off my wobbly hips, 4½ ins! Wow! It must be a combination of the exercises and diet. I have certainly changed my lifestyle. Before starting the programme, I would never have drunk so much water or eaten so many fresh foods. Looking back, I really didn't take proper care.

DAY 17 I'm feeling very positive and have 'upped' the exercise level again so I am now working up a sweat.

I got my husband to give me a massage which was very nice and ended up with us both burning off more calories!

DAY 19 Doing well. The Salad Niçoise was nice. I can't imagine having a day without exercise now, it has become so much a part of my routine. I even came home early from my friend's house, to make sure I could fit in the routine. Only another eleven days to go, but I think I will carry on repeating the programme until I get to my target weight. It would be great to weigh 10 stone.

DAY 21 I am still feeling very much in control and more positive about myself. Taking time out for myself is now something I think I am entitled to rather than feeling guilty for not doing other things instead. Even something as silly as having a bath with the door locked or going for a walk on my own seems fine now. This time is my time.

DAY 24 The children went back to school after the holidays today so I was at home. The biscuit tin was close at hand, but I wasn't tempted at all. I do enjoy the recipes; today, I used lime in cooking for the first time and the taste was delicious.

DAY 26 I went to see the hairdresser today about having a cut and possible perm. He told me that the weight of my hair meant that a sleek-looking style would be great but a perm might spoil the natural look. I'm so glad we had a long talk. I have decided to take his advice.

DAY 30 Last official day today, and I had my hair cut too. What a day! I weighed in at 10lb lighter than I was 30 days ago, and even more amazing, I have lost 7 inches off my hips. It just shows that 30 days *can* make such a difference if you want it too.

Carol repeated the programme twice, and slimmed down to 10½ stone. She is now maintaining that weight, and has decided to go on the programme again before her next holiday.

Name: **Michelle Gibson**
Age: **34** *Height*: **5ft 4in**
Starting weight: **13st 3lb**
Weight after 30 days: **12st 6lb**
Total weight loss: **11lb**
Starting measurements: **43–37–45 inches**
Measurements after 30 days: **41–32–40½ inches**

DAY 1 I've just returned from a mammoth shopping trip and am feeling very self-righteous. I've bought lots of fresh fruit and vegetables, Shape Low-Fat Soft Cheese, low-fat natural yogurt and no crisps or biscuits. I feel very determined indeed.

DAY 2 I woke up this morning and didn't feel hungry and furthermore the citrus fruit in water really woke me up. I'm used to sitting huddled in a chair waiting for the first coffee to 'kick in' but I really feel alive without it. I am still feeling positive and the exercises are fun. I certainly don't feel overstretched by them.

DAY 6 I've lost 4½lb in five days. This morning, my engagement ring is loose on my finger. I feel good about myself and have stepped up the exercises to Stage Two. They're tougher, but I feel as though I'm achieving a lot.

Enjoying the positive-thinking programme. It made me feel a bit self-centred at first, but I think my family are getting the benefit of it because I'm not nearly as ratty as normal!

DAY 8 A friend called in this morning and remarked that I looked thinner in the face. Was it the result of surgery? Hastily assured her that I am doing facial exercises every day.

I'm finding Stage Two of the exercises easier now and I think I spotted a waistline in the mirror this morning!

DAY 11 I took my daughter to a birthday party today and someone asked me if I've lost some weight. I could have kissed them! The exercises are getting easier. Tonight, I'm trying the camomile teabags in my bath. I have to say that I'm really enjoying the positive-thinking programme and 10–15 minutes of having no one making demands on my brain. I'm far more tolerant of my two-year-old.

DAY 17 I can definitely recommend the foot massage especially if your partner does it for you and it's so relaxing: better than a box of chocolates any time.

We really enjoyed the supper tonight. In fact I'm loving all the cooking. I don't feel as though I'm on a diet.

DAY 22 We've been away for the Bank Holiday weekend. I'm sorry to say that I didn't stick rigidly to the programme, but I have only eaten foods that are 'healthy', so no naughty biscuits or chocs. I couldn't wait to get home to do the exercise after being stuck on a motorway for four hours. They felt good and helped me unwind.

DAY 27 I feel sluggish today, which is a shame as I am so nearly at the end of the programme. I think I threw myself too enthusiastically into the exercises yesterday. We went out with friends today, and they noticed that I have lost weight. Very encouraging. I had my hair cut and permed. It looks brilliant, lighter and brighter and softer around my face.

When I got home I checked on the scales, I found I have *gained* 2lbs. Hope it's just a hiccup!

DAY 30 Well, this is it. I have lost quite a bit, and certainly look a whole lot better. But I am still not satisfied. I am going to carry on for another 30 days.

Michelle shed another stone, and has maintained her weight loss. She is delighted with her new look.

Name: **Sue Tucker**
Age **37** *Height*: **5ft 7in**
Starting weight: **10st**
Weight after 30 days: **9st 5lb**
Total weight loss: **9lb**
Starting measurements **34–29–39 inches**
Measurements after 30 days: **34–26–36½ inches**

DAY 1 I've started off well by doing everything according to the programme instructions, but it is only Day 1. Let's hope I can keep this enthusiasm going.

I have never been on a diet like this before. You seem to eat so much. The exercises are fairly easy, so perhaps I'm fitter than I thought.

DAY 3 Had a headache all day and found it very difficult to concentrate at work. Could this be caffeine withdrawal symptoms? I felt great otherwise and did everything. I couldn't manage to eat all the pasta at lunchtime.

DAY 6 I felt quite hungry between breakfast and lunch and a bit dizzy by lunchtime. I also got very tired on my walk, so maybe I'm not so fit after all. Dinner was excellent, but I made it cheaper by using turkey bits instead of posh chicken breasts!

DAY 11 Weighed in at 9st 6½ and felt good. I couldn't face baked beans for breakfast, so had cereal instead.

The dizziness seems to have gone, and I feel a lot better. Started doing extra exercises today, a video and some additional hip exercises. That's the bit of me that I'd like to trim down most of all.

DAY 14 I feel much firmer around the middle now. It is definitely working! Everyone liked the Tomato and Carrot Soup so much last night, that they finished it, so I had to have a tuna sandwich instead. The Budapest Pork was lovely.

DAY 15 We had friends for dinner tonight and served the Stir-Fry. They thought it was lovely. I felt a bit light-headed after doing the exercises, but I have had a couple of very late nights and am feeling rather tired.

DAY 16 Sorry, but we have to have Sunday lunch, so I couldn't follow the programme recipes. However, I just had chicken, one boiled potato and lots of vegetables. Still haven't caught up on my sleep, so I only did the set exercises and the walk, not the video. Generally feel great.

DAY 21 Went for a bike ride instead of a walk today, and I must be getting fitter because I made it all the way up a steep hill. Everyone was very impressed. My jeans are getting baggy, and I've tried on some of the skirts in my wardrobe. They look good. I really must start wearing them again. I've spent too much time in leggings and baggy tops lately.

DAY 25 I put too much cayenne pepper in the Herby Tomato Sauce so I ruined it. Never mind. I have got a bad cold, so I have only been doing the basic exercise. How can you get a cold when you are eating so much vitamin-packed food. It's a mystery! However, I weighed in and found another pound has come off. Hurrah!

DAY 27 Had my hair cut and re-shaped today. It looks super and has given me lots of confidence. The hairdresser insisted on brushing it forward, though. I think I will be going back to my 'brushed back' look again . . . it's more me! I tried on waistcoats in a shop and bought one. Just what I need to team with skirts, trousers and tops and not too expensive.

DAY 30 The cold has gone, and I feel wonderful again. I am very pleased with my weight loss. I wish I had done this five years ago. People are saying I look years younger, and I certainly never thought I would be in such good shape again. After having two children, you tend to give up. Shame! I can recommend this programme to anyone. It is wonderful. The only problem is . . . what do I do tomorrow?

Sue has maintained her weight-loss and exercise level. She looks wonderful, and at least ten years younger than her real age.

As you can see from the diary extracts above, our volunteers found the New You programme to be an interesting, rewarding experience. Like them, you will probably have 'ups and downs'. If you have problems at first such as bloating or blemishes on your skin, don't worry. Continue with the diet, exercises and beauty treatments and you will find that these minor 'blips' will vanish, leaving you feeling terrific.

You are bound to be faced with some personal worries during the 30 days. Hopefully you won't lose your job as Linda Henson did! However, even if things do go wrong, don't use this as an excuse to give up. Good nutrition and regular exercise really do help you to think positively, even if things are gloomy. Stick with it!

CHAPTER SEVEN

HOW TO BE A 'NEW YOU' FOREVER!

Once you've shaped up on the New You Programme, you will begin to enjoy all the benefits of a fitter, healthier lifestyle. You will be more energetic, have more fun and bags more confidence. So, how do you stay that way? After the first few weeks it could be very easy to slip gradually back into old, bad habits: eating the wrong foods, 'forgetting' to exercise, taking less time to do the things you want to do. So, what you need is a maintenance plan that will help you ensure that the lessons you have learned during the 30 days are not wasted.

If you have lost weight, you also need an eating programme which will allow you to 'top up' the foods to a level which keeps you at your ideal weight. In this chapter, I have set out some strategies which will achieve these objectives, a diet plan which can be adapted to suit your own particular lifestyle and metabolism, and an exercise programme which will keep you in trim.

YOUR MAINTENANCE STRATEGIES

Here are ten ways to ensure that you stay in shape:

1. Weigh in once a week and keep a record of your weight. Try the Maintenance Diet below and add extra foods until you find that your weight is steady. If you

find yourself drifting away from this eating plan, don't worry too much until your weight reaches a 5lb 'ceiling' above your New-You weight. If that happens, go back on the first seven days of menus given on the 30-day programme. If you are still too heavy, try the second seven days' menus, and so on.

Never make the mistake of crash-dieting after a calorific holiday or indulgent weekend. Yes, you will very quickly lose the weight you gained, but you will also put it on again equally quickly. You will also ruin all the health benefits gained from the holiday or weekend by starving your body of essential vitamins and minerals. It is much better to use the 30-day menus and lose the weight gradually, over a week or so, without sacrificing good nutrition.

2. Get a partner or friend to 'monitor' your shape. Most husbands, lovers or best friends will be honest enough to let you know if you are slipping back into bad habits. Ask a loved-one to be very frank with you and tell you immediately if they notice a few extra wobbly bits, or feel that you are letting yourself go a little. Once you've shrieked at them, sit down calmly and consider whether they are telling the truth. Why should they lie?

3. Practise the Body Image exercises at least once a week. Imagine yourself looking and feeling as you do now (i.e. super!) in each situation. Project forward by imagining yourself at a forthcoming party, family outing, or on next summer's holiday, in tip-top shape and form. If you do this regularly, you will help your brain 'programme' your body so that it conforms to this powerful image.

4. Walk at Stage Three for at least 20 minutes three times a week, more if you can make it. This will help 'rev up' your metabolism and encourage fat-burning.

5. Have fun. If you enjoy your new shape, you are more likely to stay in trim. So, carry on wearing those 'best' clothes, going out and about, being sociable. The more you are on show, the better.

6. Pick two kinds of exercise, and stick with them. The first kind should be sport-related, and hugely enjoyable, so you do it for fun as well as for the good of your health. Pick swimming, ice-skating, indoor tennis, basket ball, or squash. Aim to indulge in your chosen sport at least twice a week, more if you can make it. For your second exercise, choose one of the body-shaping techniques such as yoga, step-aerobics, Pilates or Nautilus. Again, you should go for the technique that you enjoy most.

7. Make time for beauty treatments. The simple beauty baths and facial treatments in Chapter Three should become part of your daily routine. If you find yourself slipping, set aside one long, lazy afternoon each week and have a facial, bath and massage as well. You deserve it.

8. Tidy your wardrobe regularly. Don't wait until the jumble of clothes, old shoes, belts and accumulated junks gets so out of control that the door will not close. Simply throw everything on the bed, and weed out the rubbish. Just getting rid of all the old wire hangers from the cleaners is a good start. Then you will be able to decide which clothes will have a new lease of life after a trip to the cleaners, and what essential item you need to buy to 'pull' a new look together.

Remember, it needn't be expensive. A super waistcoat, belt, or a piece of bold jewelry that goes with trousers, tops, shirts and skirts would be a brilliant choice.

9. Plan your life around 'treats'. The healthiest, most stress-free people are those who can create the correct balance between work, exercise, pleasure and family responsibilities. It isn't easy. So what is their secret? One business tycoon told me that his stress survival plan includes at least one self-indulgent 'treat' every day, whatever the pressures of work and family happen to be. He goes to the gym, enjoys a trip to a gallery, or has dinner with a loved-one. You can do the same. If you've worked hard, or spent a lot of time sorting out family problems, you deserve praise. You cannot count on other people to give you any (they are probably too wrapped up in their own problems), so give yourself a pat on the back instead, and reward yourself with a swim, a workout or one of the Morale Boosters on page 46.

10. Keep this book in a prominent place, not just tucked in a bookcase. I suggest you put it on your bedside table, or in the bathroom. Just catching sight of the cover each day will give you a jolt and help you stay in line. You will get a daily reminder of just how good you felt on Day 30. If you don't feel quite so good these days, it's time to repeat the programme. You can do it!

LIFETIME DIET PLAN
If you have achieved your 'happy' weight by following the programme (i.e. perfect for you, not a skinny super-model!), you can stay in shape by following the maintenance plan below.

In order to help you work out the perfect personal version of the diet, I have calculated it in calories.

The basic plan consists of menus which will provide around 1500 calories daily. There are masses of choices, so you'll never get bored! You should follow it for a week, and if you are still losing, add 100 calories daily from the Extras list on page 118. Still losing? Add another 100 calories-worth of 'Extras', and so on.

If you are a woman in a sedentary job who exercises three times a week (you do, don't you?), you'll need around 2000 calories daily. So, you should be able to indulge in five 100-calorie 'extras' daily, and stay at about the same weight. If you are a man, or very active woman, you should be able to top up your calorie intake to around 2300–2500 daily. It is really a process of trial and error. However, you are unlikely to overdo things if you stick to foods which are low in fat, high in carbohydrate and moderate in calories.

If you haven't got time for the breakfast meal (Oh yes, you have!), then choose one of the packed meal ideas and take it to work with you. It is absolutely essential to eat early in the day if you want to stay slim. Once you slip back into the habit of eating very little all day and a huge meal at night, you are doomed! Sorry!

Here is the 1500 calorie plan:

DAILY ALLOWANCES

- ½ pt (275ml) skimmed milk daily for tea, the occasional cup of coffee, and cereal.
- 1 glass dry wine or ½ pt (275ml) beer or (rarely, though!) 1 pub-measure 'double' of spirits with low-calorie mixer. *Calories*: 200

BREAKFASTS (*Choose one* – 350 calories)

- Crunchy Breakfast Special (*see* recipe on page 120)
- 1 small glass unsweetened fruit juice, Spicy Banana

on Toast (*see* recipe on page 122), Diet yogurt or fromage frais, any flavour

- Fruity Breakfast Roll (*see* recipe on page 121), 1 small glass unsweetened fruit juice, 1 apple
- Gypsy Toast (*see* recipe on page 121), grilled tomatoes, 1 rasher well-grilled lean back bacon, 2 tbsp (30ml) sweetcorn
- Nutty Orange Sunshine Breakfast (*see* recipe on page 121), 1 slice wholemeal toast with a scraping of honey or marmalade
- 1½ oz (40g) any unsweetened cereal, milk from allowance, 1 egg, boiled or poached, 1 slice wholemeal toast with scraping of low-fat spread
- 1 slice wholemeal toast topped with 1 small can (5oz/150g) baked beans, grilled tomatoes, 1 small glass unsweetened fruit juice, 1 apple or pear
- 1 sandwich of 2 slices wholemeal bread with one of the following fillings: 1 rasher well-grilled lean bacon, sliced tomatoes, lettuce OR 2 tbsp (30ml) cottage cheese with pineapple, ½ oz (15g) chopped lean ham OR 1 medium banana, mashed with 2 tbsp (30ml) low-fat natural yogurt and a sprinkling of cinnamon. Plus 1 apple, orange or small banana

MID-MORNING (*Choose one* – 50 calories)

- 1 apple, orange, pear, nectarine, peach or small banana
- 2 crispbreads with scraping of Shape Low-Fat Soft Cheese, sliced tomatoes and watercress
- 1 digestive biscuit

LUNCH (*Choose one* – 350 calories)

- Vegetable and Pasta Salad (*see* recipe on page 146), 1 slice wholemeal bread, 1 apple or orange

- 4 crispbreads with one serving Smoked Mackerel Pâté (*See* recipe on page 127), mixed salad with lemon-juice dressing, 1 diet yogurt (any flavour), 1 medium banana
- Melon and Cottage Cheese Salad (*see* recipe on page 122), 1 medium wholemeal roll with 1 tbsp (15ml) Shape Low-Fat Soft Cheese, a few grapes
- Fruity Open Sandwich (*see* recipe on page 125), 1 medium glass tomato juice, or V8 vegetable juice
- Tomato and Carrot Soup (*see* recipe on page 148), a sandwich of 2 slices wholemeal bread with salad and 2oz (50g) cooked chicken (no skin)
- 1 sandwich of 2 slices wholemeal bread or large wholemeal roll with one of these fillings and extras: Mexican Tuna (*see* recipe on page 126), a few grapes *OR* 1oz (25g) lean ham, 1 small banana *OR* 1oz (25g) grated low-fat cheese mixed with 1 dsp (10ml) low-calorie mayonnaise, 2 sticks celery
- 1 mug Batchelors Slim a Soup, 1 pitta bread with filling of salad and 2oz (50g) cooked chicken (no skin) *OR* 3oz (75g) tuna canned in brine, and 1 apple, pear, orange, nectarine or peach

MID-AFTERNOON (*Choose one* – 100 calories)

- 1 medium banana
- 1 packet low-fat crisps (yes, really!)
- 1 apple, orange, pear, nectarine or peach plus 1 small digestive biscuit or 2 crispbreads with a scraping of Shape Low-Fat Soft Cheese
- 1 mug Batchelors Slim a Soup or an Ovaltine Options Chocolate-flavour drink and 1 crispbread with a scraping of Marmite, jam or honey

SUPPER (*Choose one* – 450 calories)

- Gammon Steak with Pineapple and Mustard Sauce (*see* recipe on page 134), 8oz (225g) jacket potato, cauliflower, courgettes, 2 tbsp (30ml) sweetcorn, 1 medium banana
- Slice of melon, Lamb Chops with Orange and Mint Sauce (*see* recipe on page 134), 3oz (75g) boiled potatoes, broccoli, green beans, grilled tomatoes, huge mixed salad with lemon-juice dressing
- Stir Fried Chicken (*see* recipe on page 136), 3 tbsp (45ml) wholegrain rice, huge mixed salad with lemon-juice dressing, 1 pear with ½oz (12.5g) low-fat hard cheese
- Spaghetti with Ham and Cheese Sauce (*see* recipe on page 140), tomato, cucumber, basil and sliced onion salad with 1 dsp (10ml) Kraft Fat Free Vinaigrette Style Dressing, a few grapes
- Chicken and Corn Casserole (*see* recipe on page 133), 2oz (50g) potato, mashed with milk from allowance, cabbage, cauliflower, 2 tbsp (30ml) carrots, baked apple with 1 tsp (5ml) honey and a few raisins
- Budapest Pork (*see* recipe on page 132), courgettes, green beans, red cabbage, 1 diet yogurt or fromage frais, any flavour
- Prawn and Mushroom Risotto (*see* recipe on page 130), huge mixed salad with lemon-juice dressing, medium banana baked in foil with 1 tsp (5ml) honey and served with 1 dsp (10ml) fromage frais
- Bangers with Rice (*see* recipe on page 131), grilled tomatoes, watercress
- Cod in a Parcel (*see* recipe on page 129), 10oz (275g) jacket potato, broccoli, courgettes, 2 tbsp (30ml) peas, 1oz (25g) scoop vanilla icecream with sauce made from 2 tsp (10ml) jam and a little hot water

- 3oz (75g) any lean roast meat, thin gravy, 3oz (75g) large chunks roast potato, cauliflower, courgettes, 2 tbsp (30ml) carrots, 2 tbsp (30ml) peas, 1 diet yogurt or fromage frais
- 1 well-grilled beefburger, 1 small can (5oz/125g) baked beans, grilled tomatoes, watercress, 3oz (75g) oven chips, lettuce, cucumber, 1 wholemeal roll

Eating Out At a carvery, choose melon or clear soup to start, turkey or chicken, lots of vegetables and a water ice for dessert. Avoid thick gravy, chips and fatty meat. At an Indian restaurant, go for Chicken Tikka or Tandoori, plain boiled rice and a side salad. At a Chinese Restaurant, choose a Chicken Chop Suey and plain boiled rice. Avoid anything covered in batter. If you are going Italian, choose the cold starter with seafood and salad, and plain pasta with a tomato sauce. No cream, sorry.

EXTRAS (Select according to the instructions above – they are all around 100 calories)

- 1 slice wholemeal bread or small wholemeal roll
- 1 extra glass of wine or beer
- 1 medium banana or 2 apples, oranges, pears, nectarines or peaches
- 1 'fun size' Mars, Marathon or Snickers Bar
- 1 small packet low-fat crisps
- 1 small carton cottage cheese or natural, unsweetened yogurt
- 1 diet yogurt, any flavour, with 1 apple, orange or small banana
- 2oz (50g) lean ham or chicken (no skin) *OR* 4oz (100g) portion grilled fish *OR* 2oz (50g) portion red meat (no skin or gristle)

BASIC EXERCISE PROGRAMME

If you follow this plan, you will maintain your trim shape and feel just great.

EVERY DAY

1. Complete Breath
2. Complete Posture Programme
3. Problem area exercises: concentrate on the areas where fat is most likely to build up. For instance, bottom, hips and thighs, tummy. Exercise those areas every day. In addition, choose exercises which are suitable for your own figure, adding those to your programme two or three times a week.
4. Wind Down exercise.

THREE TIMES A WEEK

Walking Go for Stage Three level walking. You know you enjoy it! Seriously, it will really help to keep you trim and can easily be fitted into the busiest schedule if you combine it with other activities like shopping, walking the dog, or just dashing from home to work.

TWICE A WEEK

Sport Fit in your own personal sporting regime, using the ideas in Number 6 of the Maintenance Strategies on page 112. Swimming is an easy one, before work or at lunchtime. Squash is a great 'wind down' exercise after work, and skating is fun at weekends.

Body Shaping Go to a class locally. There are now so many excellent fitness clubs running regular classes that it should be easy to find a yoga session or step aerobics session that will neatly slot into your routine.

CHAPTER EIGHT

RECIPES FOR HEALTHY GOOD LOOKS

Here are all the recipes you need for the New You programme. They have all been calorie-counted and quantities are given in imperial and metric measurements – work in either, but *not* both.

BREAKFASTS

CRUNCHY BREAKFAST SPECIAL

8oz (225g) rolled oats
2oz (50g) wheatgerm
4oz (100g) small dried apricots, chopped
6oz (175g) sultanas
2oz (50g) walnuts, roughly chopped
½ pear or apple (per portion), peeled, cored and grated
1 level tsp (5ml) honey (per portion)
3 level tbsp (30ml) natural, low-fat yogurt (per portion)

1. Mix the dry fruit and cereal together. Store in an airtight container.

2. For breakfast, add grated apple or pear to each portion, top with yogurt and dribble with honey.

Serves: 8   *Calories per serving*: 340

FRUITY BREAKFAST ROLL

1 crusty wholemeal roll
1 apple, cored and chopped
½ oz (15g) raisins
1 tbsp (15ml) lemon juice
1 level tbsp (15ml) cottage cheese or low-fat fromage frais

1. Split the roll.

2. Mix remaining ingredients together and pile onto one half. Place the second half on top, and munch!

Serves: 1   *Calories per serving*: 235

GYPSY TOAST

1 size 3 egg
1 slice wholemeal bread
salt and black pepper

1. Place egg in a shallow dish and beat well.

2. Soak bread in the egg then fry quickly without added fat in a non-stick pan.

Serves: 1   *Calories per serving*: 170

NUTTY ORANGE SUNSHINE BREAKFAST

1 large orange
1 apple, peeled, cored and chopped
1 level dsp (10ml) raisins
1 level dsp (10ml) chopped dates
1 level dsp (10ml) pine kernels or mixed chopped nuts
2 level tbsp (30ml) fromage frais

1. Halve the orange, scoop out the flesh, keeping shells intact.

2. Chop flesh, removing pith, and place in a bowl.

3. Add the chopped apple, raisins and nuts. Pile back into orange shells and top with fromage frais.

Serves: 2   *Calories per serving*: 115

SPICY BANANA ON TOAST

1 small ripe banana
1 level tbsp (15ml) natural, low-fat yogurt
1 level tsp (5ml) apricot or strawberry jam
pinch of ground cinnamon
1 slice wholemeal bread

1. Mash banana, yogurt and jam together

2. Add a pinch of ground cinnamon and spread on a slice of wholemeal toast.

Serves: 1   *Calories per serving*: 185

LUNCHES

SALADS

MELON AND COTTAGE CHEESE SALAD

1 medium melon, cut in half around the circumference
  and deseeded
2oz (50g) lean ham, chopped
2 sticks celery, chopped
2oz (50g) button mushrooms, sliced
½ cucumber, deseeded and diced
1 tbsp (15ml) lemon juice
4oz (100g) cottage cheese
paprika and sprigs of watercress to decorate

1. Cut melon flesh into balls with a teaspoon and place in a bowl with ham, celery, mushrooms and cucumber.

2. Mix well, then pour over lemon juice and fold in yogurt.

3. Put back into the melon halves and pile the cottage cheese on top. Decorate with pinch of paprika and watercress sprigs.

Serves: 2   *Calories per serving*: 150

PASTA WALDORF SALAD

3oz (75g) cooked pasta shapes
3oz (75g) cucumber unpeeled
2 sticks celery
1oz (25g) onion,
2½ fl oz (70ml) natural low-fat yogurt
1 level tbsp (15ml) low-calorie mayonnaise
garlic and celery salt to taste
1 medium red apple, unpeeled
lemon juice

1. Place pasta in a basin.

2. Chop cucumber, celery and onion and add to pasta.

3. Mix yogurt with seasoning and mayonnaise and pour over pasta and vegetables.

4. Toss and place on a plate, or in a sealed container to take to work.

5. Just before eating, wash and dice apple, toss in lemon juice and pile on top of the salad.

Serves: 1   *Calories per serving*: 275

SANDWICHES, TOPPINGS AND FILLINGS

CHEESY FISH GRILL

1 thick slice wholemeal bread
1½oz (40g) any cooked smoked fish (e.g. haddock,
  mackerel)
1oz (25g) onion, finely sliced
1 medium tomato, sliced
salt and freshly ground black pepper
1oz (25g) low-fat hard cheese, grated

1. Toast bread on one side.

2. Place fish on the other side, cover with onion rings,
tomato and season.

3. Top with grated cheese and grill slowly until cheese
is melted.

Serves: 1   *Calories per serving*: 230, using smoked had-
              dock, 345 using smoked mackerel

EASTERN PITTA TREAT

1 wholemeal pitta bread
½ small avocado pear, peeled and chopped and sprin-
  kled with lemon juice to prevent discolouration
2oz (50g) cooked chicken or turkey, cut into strips
  (no skin)
1 tomato, peeled, deseeded and chopped

Dressing
1oz (25g) Shape Soft Cheese
juice ½ small lemon
salt and pepper
1 tsp (5ml) chopped chives

1. Cut pitta bread in half and open out the 'pocket' with a knife.

2. Mix the filling ingredients, toss lightly in the dressing and stuff into the pitta pocket.

Serves: 1   *Calories per serving*: 400

FRUITY OPEN SANDWICH

1 slice wholemeal bread (1¼oz/35g)
1 large lettuce leaf
1½oz (40g) sliced lean cooked pork or ham
2oz (50g) low-calorie coleslaw salad
1 kiwi fruit, peeled and sliced
4 cashew nuts

1. Top the slice of bread with the lettuce leaf and meat.

2. Spoon over the coleslaw and garnish with kiwi fruit slices and cashew nuts.

Serves: 1   *Calories per serving*: 245

HERBY TOMATO SAUCE

3 small onions or shallots, finely chopped
2 cloves of garlic, peeled and crushed
pinch of cayenne pepper
6 fl oz (175ml) chicken stock
6 fl oz (175ml) dry red or white wine
1 tbsp (15ml) fresh chopped parsley
1 tbsp each chopped fresh basil, thyme and oregano or ¼
    level tsp (1.25ml) each dried basil, thyme and oregano
3 cans (14oz/397g) chopped tomatoes
salt and freshly-ground black pepper
2 level tbsp (30ml) tomato paste

1. Combine onion, garlic, cayenne, stock, wine and herbs in a heavy frying pan. Bring to the boil, reduce heat and simmer briskly until almost all the liquid has been evaporated.

2. Stir in the drained tomatoes, chopping roughly with a wooden spatula.

3. Season, and simmer uncovered for 15 minutes.

4. Stir in the tomato paste, simmer for a further 5 minutes and serve.

Serves: 4   *Calories per serving*: 105

MEXICAN TUNA

6oz (175g) tuna, canned in brine
¼ green pepper, deseeded and chopped or 2oz (50g)
   button mushrooms, sliced
2oz (50g) canned sweetcorn, drained
3½oz (90g) canned kidney beans, drained
dash of Tabasco and lemon juice

Mix all ingredients in a bowl and use as a sandwich or pitta bread filler.

Serves: 2   *Calories per serving*: 170

PRAWN COCKTAIL SANDWICH FILLING

1oz (25g) peeled prawns
1dsp (10ml) low-fat natural yogurt
1 level tsp (5ml) low-calorie mayonnaise
¼ tsp (1.25ml) tomato ketchup
1 drop Tabasco sauce

Combine ingredients in a small bowl and use to fill a sandwich or roll.

Serves: 1   *Calories per serving*: 55, plus approximately 150 for bread or roll

SALMON PÂTÉ

4oz (100g) canned red salmon, drained
4oz (100g) reduced-fat Cheddar type cheese, finely grated
2 tsps (10ml) lemon juice
1 tsp (5ml) Worcestershire sauce
2 level tbsp (30ml) low-calorie mayonnaise
grated rind of 1 small lemon
1 tbsp (15ml) parsley, finely chopped
1 level tbsp (15ml) chopped nuts

Beat all the ingredients together, place on a serving dish and chill.

Serves: 4   *Calories per serving*: 155

SMOKED MACKEREL PÂTÉ

3oz (75g) smoked mackerel, skinned
2oz (50g) Shape Low-Fat Soft Cheese
2 level tbsp (30ml) natural, low-fat yogurt
lemon juice

Skin and flake mackerel and place in a blender with soft cheese and lemon juice.

Serves: 2   *Calories per serving*: 200

SPICY TOMATO JUICE DRESSING

4 tbsp (60ml) tomato juice
4 tbsp (60ml) wine vinegar
1 tsp (5ml) Worcestershire sauce
2 tsp (10ml) finely chopped shallots or spring onions

½ level tsp (2.5ml) dried basil
freshly ground black pepper and salt to taste

Shake all ingredients together in a screw-topped jar.

Serves: 4   *Calories per serving*: 5

SPINACH AND SOFT CHEESE PÂTÉ

150g carton Philadelphia Light or Shape Soft Cheese
4oz (100g) frozen spinach
a few drops of Tabasco
juice of ½ lemon
grated nutmeg
salt and pepper
4 lemon twists to garnish

1. Beat the cream cheese until soft.

2. Cook and drain the spinach thoroughly, then gradually add to the soft cheese, beating constantly.

3. Add the Tabasco, lemon juice, nutmeg and seasoning to taste.

4. Spoon into four individual dishes and chill. Garnish each portion with a twist of lemon.

Serves: 4   *Calories per serving*: 55 using Shape, 80 using Philadelphia Light

SUPPERS

DESSERT

RED FRUIT SUNDAE

1lb (450g) mixed 'red' fruits – plums, frozen
    raspberries, strawberries, nectarines etc.
2oz (50g) bran flakes
8 level tbsp (120ml) diet fromage frais, fruit flavoured

1. Chop fruit into bite-sized pieces and divide between
four sundae glasses.

2. Sprinkle with crushed bran flakes and chill.

3. Serve with 1 rounded tbsp (15ml) fromage frais on
each sundae.

Serves: 4   *Calories per serving*: 100

FISH

COD IN A PARCEL

4 cod fillets, about 4oz (100g) each
2 tbsp (30 ml) chopped fresh parsley
4tbsp (60ml) chopped fresh mint
4 tbsp (60ml) lemon juice
4 tbsp (60ml) dry white wine
salt and freshly ground black pepper

1. Place each cod fillet on a large square of foil.
Sprinkle parsley, mint, lemon juice and wine on top and
season.

2. Fold up foil neatly to make loose parcels with tightly
sealed edges, and bake in a hot oven (180°C, 350°F,
Gas Mark 4) for about 30 minutes.

3. Serve each parcel slightly undone to release the aroma of herbs, wine and lemon juice.

Serves: 4 *Calories per serving*: 100

PRAWN AND MUSHROOM RISOTTO

1 tsp (5ml) oil
¼ oz (7g) butter
1 small onion, finely chopped
1 clove garlic, finely chopped
pinch turmeric or mild curry powder
4oz (100g) risotto or long-grain white rice
12fl oz (350ml) fish stock, from cube
4oz (100g) mushrooms, sliced
1oz (25g) frozen sweetcorn
4oz (100g) peeled prawns
salt and pepper to taste
freshly chopped parsley and lemon wedges to
  garnish

1. Heat the oil and butter in a non-stick frying pan and cook onion until transparent.

2. Add garlic and turmeric, stir briefly to blend with the onion.

3. Add rice and stir for two or three minutes.

4. Then add sweetcorn, stock, and seasoning.

5. Simmer, covered, for about 20 minutes, or until liquid is nearly absorbed. Stir occasionally and add a little extra stock if necessary to prevent sticking.

6. Add the mushrooms and prawns and cook for another 5 minutes.

7. Stir, test for seasoning and garnish with chopped parsley and lemon wedges.

Serves: 4   *Calories per serving*: 185

MEAT

BACON STEAKS WITH PINEAPPLE AND CHEESE TOPPING

4 gammon steaks, about 3½ oz (90g) each, with fat
   removed
2oz (50g) Shape soft cheese
1 level tbsp (15ml) chopped fresh parsley
1 clove garlic, crushed
salt and black pepper
4 slices pineapple, fresh or canned (in juice)chopped,
   or 1 orange, peeled and chopped
parsley for garnish

1. Grill the bacon steaks on both sides until beginning to brown.

2. Mix the cheese, herbs and seasoning and spread on top of the cooked steaks. Return to the grill, and cook for a few minutes until bubbly.

3. Serve garnished with chopped pineapple and parsley.

Serves: 2   *Calories per serving*: 290

BANGERS WITH RICE

4oz (100g) onion, chopped
12oz (350g) canned chopped tomatoes
1 clove garlic, crushed
oregano to taste

12oz (350g) low-fat beef or pork sausages
6oz (175g) hot, cooked fluffy rice

1. Cook the onions and tomatoes over a gentle heat in a non-stick pan until onions are soft.

2. Add garlic and oregano, bring to the boil and simmer for 15 minutes or until reduced to a thick sauce.

3. Meanwhile, grill bangers until cooked through and brown.

4. To serve, place sausages on a bed of rice and pour the sauce over the top.

Serves: 2   *Calories per serving*: 435

BUDAPEST PORK

1lb (450g) lean shoulder or leg of pork, trimmed of all
    fat and cut into small cubes
2 level tbsp (30ml) paprika
freshly ground black pepper
2 large onions, finely sliced
14oz (400g) can chopped tomatoes
2 level tbsp (30ml) tomato purée
1 pint (575ml) vegetable stock
1½ lb (675g) unpeeled potatoes, washed and diced
4oz (100g) button mushrooms, halved
5 fl oz (150ml) natural low-fat yogurt
grated rind of ½ lemon
2 tbsp (30ml) chopped parsley

1 Toss pork in the paprika and season with black pepper.

2. Put the onions in a large, non-stick saucepan and add 3 tbsp (45ml) cold water. Cover with a tight-fitting lid and cook gently for 5 minutes.

3. Remove lid, increase the heat and cook the onions briskly, stirring continuously for 2 minutes.

4. Stir in the pork, tomatoes, tomato purée and stock. Cover and simmer gently for 40 minutes.

5. Add the potatoes, cook for a further 10 minutes, adding extra stock if needed.

6. Add the mushrooms and cook for another 10 minutes.

7. Season to taste, pour into a serving dish and top with the natural yogurt, lemon rind and parsley.

Serves: 4   *Calories per serving*: 340

CHICKEN AND CORN CASSEROLE

8 part-boned chicken breasts (about 6oz/175g each)
2 x 7oz (200g) cans sweetcorn, drained
2 medium onions, sliced
15oz (425g) can chopped tomatoes
1 pint (575ml) water
1 chicken stock cube
chicken seasoning
2 level tbsp (30ml) cornflour
chopped parsley for garnish

1. Grill the chicken pieces for 5 minutes on each side, remove and discard skin.

2. Place sweetcorn, onion, tomatoes and juice, water, stock cube and seasoning in a large saucepan. Bring to the boil and simmer for 5 minutes.

3. Place chicken pieces in a large casserole dish and

pour the sauce over. Check seasoning. Cover and cook at 180°C, 350°F, Gas Mark 4 for 45 minutes.

4. Mix the cornflour with a little cold water and stir into the casserole. Cook for a further 15 minutes.

5. Serve garnished with chopped parsley.

Serves: 8   *Calories per serving*: 240

GAMMON STEAK WITH PINEAPPLE AND MUSTARD SAUCE

4 x 3oz (75g) lean gammon steaks, trimmed of fat
4 pineapple rings (canned in juice)
½ level tsp (2.5ml) made-up mustard
½ level tsp (2.5ml) yeast extract
salt and black pepper
2 tbsp (10ml) chopped parsley
parsley sprigs to garnish

1. Drain pineapple rings and reserve juice.

2. Place the gammon steaks in a shallow ovenproof dish and top each one with a pineapple ring.

3. Mix together the remaining ingredients and reserved pineapple juice and pour over the gammon and pineapple. Cook in a moderate oven (325°F, 170°C, Gas Mark 3) for 30 minutes.

4. Garnish with parsley sprigs.

Serves: 2   *Calories per serving*: 225

LAMB CHOPS WITH ORANGE AND MINT SAUCE

4 lamb loin chops, trimmed, approx 4oz (100g) each
4 fl oz (100ml) unsweetened orange juice
1 tsp (5ml) oil
4 tsp (20ml) finely chopped mint
sprigs of mint and orange slices to garnish

1. Place lamb in a shallow ovenproof dish.

2. Mix orange juice, oil and chopped mint and pour over the lamb. Marinade in the fridge for an hour.

3. Place dish under the grill and cook lamb chops until crisp on the outside but a little pink inside, basting with the marinade from time to time.

4. Serve garnished with sprigs of mint and orange slices.

Serves: 4   *Calories per serving*: 225

LAMB OR PORK KEBABS WITH BARBECUE SAUCE

1 lb (450g) lean boneless leg of lamb or pork tenderloin
1 large red pepper, cored and de-seeded
1 large green pepper, cored and de-seeded
4oz (100g) button mushrooms
8oz (225g) cherry tomatoes
oil for brushing

1. Cut the meat into cubes, discarding any fat or gristle.

2. Cut the peppers into squares.

3. Thread the meat, peppers, mushrooms and tomatoes onto skewers. Brush with oil and grill under a preheated

grill, turning frequently, until the meat is cooked through and tender.

Barbecue Sauce

1 clove garlic, crushed
1 small onion, chopped
1 small can (8oz/227g) chopped tomatoes
3 level tbsp (45ml) tomato ketchup
1 level tsp (5ml) French mustard
1 tbsp (15ml) each of bottled brown fruity sauce,
    Worcestershire sauce and soya sauce
½ pt (275ml) hot water
½ beef stock cube
seasoning
1 level tbsp (15 ml) soft brown sugar

1. Place the garlic, onion and canned tomatoes in a saucepan. Cook gently until onion is soft.

2. Add ketchup, mustard, sauces and sugar.

3. Dissolve the stock cube in the hot water and add to the saucepan. Simmer for 5 minutes.

4. Purée in a blender, then season and sweeten to taste.

Serves: 4   *Calories per serving*: 240

STIR-FRIED CHICKEN

Marinade
1 small onion, peeled and chopped
2 tbsp (30ml) soya sauce
2 tbsp (30ml) dry white wine
2 tbsp (30ml) honey
4 tbsp (60ml) water
¼ tsp (1.25ml) each of cayenne pepper and ground ginger

Main ingredients
1lb (450g) boneless skinned chicken breasts cut into cubes
2 tsp (10ml) oil
1 large red and 1 large green pepper, deseeded and
    cut into 1in squares
16 button mushrooms, sliced
2oz (50g) bean sprouts
4 spring onions, chopped
5 fl oz (150ml) Shape Single

1. Mix marinade ingredients together, stir in the chicken and leave for 1 hour.

2. Remove chicken and brown in a wok or non-stick frying pan, over a high heat for 3–4 minutes, stirring constantly.

3. Remove from the pan and keep warm.

4. Add the oil, toss the pepper, mushrooms, beansprouts and spring onion for 1 minute.

5. Return chicken to the pan and pour in the marinade. Bring to the boil.

6. Stir in the Single, heat but do not boil and check seasoning. Serve immediately.

Serves: 4   *Calories per serving*: 280

STIR-FRIED VEGETABLES WITH CHICKEN OR PORK

1tbsp (15ml) oil
1 large onion, peeled and chopped
2 carrots, cut into fine matchsticks
1in piece fresh root ginger, peeled and finely chopped
1 clove garlic, finely chopped

10oz (275g) chicken breast or pork fillet, cut into fine strips
8oz (225g) Chinese leaves or cabbage, finely sliced
3½ oz (100g) mushrooms, sliced
8oz (225g) bean-sprouts
1 tbsp (15ml) dry sherry
2 tbsp (30ml) soya sauce

1. Heat the oil in a wok or large non-stick pan and stir fry the onions, carrots and ginger for 3 minutes, stirring continuously.

2. Add the garlic and stir for another minute.

3. Remove the vegetables from the pan and fry the meat for 3 minutes, turning continously

4. Return vegetables to the pan with the cabbage or Chinese leaves, mushrooms and beansprouts and stir-fry for 2 minutes.

5. Add the sherry and soya sauce, then cover and cook for 4 minutes.

Serves: 4   *Calories per serving*: 190

SWEET AND SOUR PORK FILLET

1½ lb (675g) pork fillet
1 x 15oz (425g) can beansprouts, drained
2 tbsp (30ml) soya sauce
black pepper to taste

For the sauce

1½ tbsp (22ml) each of wine vinegar and lemon juice
4 level tbsp (60ml) tomato purée

1 level tsp (5ml) paprika
10 fl oz (275ml) water
3oz (75g) carrots, cut into fine strips
3oz (75g) green pepper, finely sliced
2 level tbsp (30ml) sugar

1. Cut pork into cubes and grill on a sheet of foil, turning frequently.

2. Place on a serving dish and keep hot.

3. Mix soya sauce, beansprouts and black pepper, and heat through in a small pan, stirring constantly. Turn into a serving dish, cover and keep hot.

4. Combine sauce ingredients and simmer for 15 minutes. Pour over pork and serve with beansprouts.

Serves: 4   *Calories per serving*: 275

PASTA

PASTA WITH GREEN BEANS AND PRAWNS

1½ lb (675g) French beans, fresh or frozen
8oz (225g) peeled prawns
8oz (225g) pasta, dry weight
1 tbsp (15ml) oil
2 cloves garlic, crushed
3 tbsp (45ml) soya sauce

1. If beans are fresh, cut them in half and cook for 5 minutes in boiling water (or until just tender). Cook frozen beans according to instructions.

2. Meanwhile, cook pasta in boiling water for 10–12 minutes. Drain.

3. Heat the oil in a non-stick pan and stir fry prawns and garlic for 2 minutes.

4. Add beans and pasta, stir for 4 minutes.

5. Sprinkle over soya sauce and serve.

Serves: 4   *Calories per serving*: 340

PASTA WITH FRESH TOMATO SAUCE

8oz (225g) (dry weight) pasta
2lb (900g) very ripe tomatoes, skinned and chopped or
    1½ lb (675g) canned tomatoes
2 level tsps (10ml) finely grated root ginger
black pepper
3 level tbsp (45ml) grated parmesan cheese

1. Gently heat the tomatoes and ginger in a non-stick pan, adding a little water if necessary. Cook over low heat for about 10 minutes.

2. Cook pasta in plenty of boiling water, drain and serve with the sauce and a little grated parmesan.

Serves: 4   *Calories per serving*: 260

SPAGHETTI WITH HAM AND CHEESE SAUCE

1 large onion, chopped
14oz (400g) can chopped tomatoes
2 garlic cloves, chopped
1 bay leaf
1 tbsp (15ml) fresh chopped basil
1 tbsp (15ml) olive oil
1 tbsp (15ml) dry white wine
¼ pt (150ml) water
½ chicken stock cube

freshly ground black pepper
4oz (100g) Shape Soft Cheese
4oz (100g) thin ham or prosciutto, lean only, cut into
   strips
10oz (275g) wholewheat, green or plain spaghetti

1. Saute the onion, garlic and bay leaf in oil until soft.

2. Add the tomatoes, wine, basil, water and stock cube.
Bring to the boil and then simmer for 10 minutes.

3. Season and stir in the soft cheese until it melts. Add
the ham.

4. Meanwhile, cook the spaghetti in boiling salted water
for about 10 minutes, until tender but not soft. Drain.

5. Serve immediately with hot sauce poured over.

Serves: 4   *Calories per serving*: 405

SPINACH NOODLES

1 onion, chopped
1oz (25g) butter
8oz (225g) frozen spinach, thawed and chopped
5oz (150g) carton natural low-fat yogurt
4oz (100g) low-fat soft cheese
1 tsp (5ml) lemon juice
salt and black pepper
¼ level tsp (1.25ml) ground nutmeg
8oz (225g) noodles

1. Saute the onion in the butter until soft.

2. Add the spinach and cook for 2 minutes.

3. Stir in the yogurt, cheese, lemon juice, seasoning and
nutmeg.

4. Meanwhile, cook the noodles in boiling water for 5 minutes. Drain. Add the spinach sauce, toss lightly and serve.

Serves: 4   *Calories per serving*: 350

SALADS

BROWN RICE AND TUNA SALAD

1 onion, chopped
1 clove garlic, crushed
1 tbsp (15ml) sunflower oil
6oz (175g) cooked brown rice (raw weight)
1oz (25g) cashew nuts
7oz (198g) can tuna fish, drained
6oz (175g) tomatoes, peeled, deseeded and chopped
6oz (175g) cucumber, diced
2oz (50g) natural low-fat yogurt
2 level tsp (10ml) French mustard

1. Saute the onion and garlic in the oil for a few minutes to soften. Cool.

2. Mix the onion with the rice, cashew nuts, tuna, 2 tomatoes, cucumber and chopped parsley.

3. Blend the natural yogurt and mustard together and pour over the rice, stirring in well. Taste and season well.

4. Serve with a leafy green salad.

Serves: 4   *Calories per serving*: 305

CELERY, PINEAPPLE AND WALNUT SALAD

4 sticks celery, chopped
12oz (350g) fresh pineapple (or canned in juice), cubed
1lb (450g) apples, cored and diced
2oz (50g) walnut pieces
2oz (50g) low-calorie mayonnaise
1 tbsp (15ml) chopped parsley
salt and black pepper

1. Mix the celery, pineapple, apple and walnuts together.

2. Coat with the mayonnaise and sprinkle with parsley.

3. Season well.

4. Chill before serving.

Serves: 4   *Calories per serving*: 205

CHICKEN SALAD SUPREME

12oz (350g) cooked chicken breasts, skinned
¼ cucumber
4 tomatoes
1 apple
juice of ½ lemon
1 level dsp (10ml) mild or wholegrain mustard
sprig of parsley or dill
2 level tbsp (30ml) low-calorie mayonnaise
2 tsp (10ml) wine vinegar
1 tbsp (15ml) orange juice
1 level tsp (5ml) grated orange rind

1. Skin the chicken and carve the meat into thin slices.

2. Wash and dry the cucumber, cut in half lengthwise, scoop out the seeds and slice finely.

3. Peel and halve tomatoes. Remove seeds and dice the flesh.

4. Peel, quarter and core the apple and sprinkle with the lemon juice.

5. Mix chicken, cucumber, tomatoes and apple together in a bowl.

6. Beat the mustard into the mayonnaise.

7. Wash and finely chop the parsley or dill.

8. Mix the vinegar and orange juice together and stir into the mayonnaise with the parsley or dill and grated orange rind.

9. Arrange the salad on four dishes and divide the dressing between the portions.

Serves: 4   *Calories per serving*: 195

MUSHROOM AND BEANSPROUT SALAD

12oz (350g) button mushrooms, quartered
6 tbsp (90ml) Kraft Fat Free Vinaigrette Style
   Dressing
8oz (225g) beansprouts, fresh or canned, drained
1 red pepper, cored, seeded and finely chopped

1. Place mushrooms in a bowl, add the dressing and toss well.

2. Marinade for 1 hour.

3. Then add beansprouts and pepper. Toss thoroughly.

Serves: 4   *Calories per serving*: 45

ORANGE AND WATERCRESS SALAD

1 bunch watercress
2 large oranges
juice of ½ lemon

1. Wash watercress, remove stalks and place in a large salad bowl.

2. Cut off both ends of each orange with a sharp knife. Remove skin and pith and slice into thin rounds with a bread knife. Cut each slice into quarters, remove pips and toss with the watercress and lemon juice.

Serves: 2   *Calories per serving*: 80

SALAD NIÇOISE

1 large head of lettuce such as Webbs or Iceberg
4 large ripe tomatoes, sliced
8oz (225g) French beans or runner beans, cooked
3 tbsp (45ml) Kraft Fat Free Vinaigrette Style
   Dressing
7oz (200g) tuna canned in brine, drained
2oz (50g) can anchovies in oil, drained
2 eggs, hard-boiled and halved
12 black olives

1. Wash and dry lettuce and place in a large salad bowl.

2. Add the tomatoes, beans and dressing and gently mix together.

3. Arrange remaining ingredients on top of the salad.

Serves: 4   *Calories per serving*: 245

VEGETABLE AND PASTA SALAD

8oz (225g) wholemeal pasta spirals
4oz (100g) cherry tomatoes
8oz (225g) small button mushrooms
6 large black olives
1 tbsp (15ml) finely chopped coriander or parsley
4 level tbsp (60ml) Kraft Fat Free Vinaigrette Style
  Dressing

1. Cook pasta spirals in boiling salted water until firm but not soft.

2. Halve cherry tomatoes and mushrooms, finely chop olives.

3. Drain pasta, mix everything together and keep in refrigerator until required.

Serves: 4   *Calories per serving*: 200

SOUPS

GAZPACHO

1 large cucumber
1 medium green pepper, cored and deseeded
1 medium red pepper, cored and deseeded
1–3 cloves garlic, chopped
1 tbsp (15ml) wine vinegar
1½ pt (850ml) tomato juice, chilled
7oz (200g) can chopped tomatoes, chilled
juice of ½ lemon
salt and black pepper

1. Cut half the cucumber and the peppers into tiny cubes and arrange on a serving dish as garnish.

2. Roughly chop the remaining cucumber and peppers. Put in a blender with the garlic and wine vinegar and liquidize until smooth.

3. Stir into chilled tomato juice.

4. Finally, stir in the chilled, chopped tomatoes and lemon juice and season.

5. Serve in a large bowl with ice cubes, and the garnish separately.

Serves: 4   *Calories per serving*: 65

LEEK AND POTATO SOUP

1 tbsp (15ml) sunflower oil
3 leeks, washed and sliced
10oz (275g) potatoes, peeled
1pt (575ml) chicken stock
salt and pepper
1 level tbsp (15ml) mixed herbs
pinch of paprika pepper
¼ pt (150ml) Shape Double
4 tbsp (60ml) Shape Single or natural, unsweetened
   yogurt
1 tbsp (15ml) chopped chives

1. Heat the oil in a large pan, add the vegetables and cook for a few minutes.

2. Stir in the stock and season. Cover and simmer for 30 minutes until the potatoes are tender.

3. Add the Double and liquidize or sieve the soup.

4. Chill if you are serving it cold (luscious!) or heat through if you prefer it hot. Serve in four bowls

garnished with a swirl of Single or natural yogurt and chopped chives.

Serves: 4   *Calories per serving*: 215

TOMATO AND CARROT SOUP

4oz (100g) carrots, peeled and sliced
2oz (50g) onion, chopped
1 clove garlic, chopped
1 tbsp (15ml) sunflower oil
1 lb (450g) fresh ripe tomatoes, chopped
1 pint (575ml) chicken stock
salt and pepper
a little grated nutmeg
1oz (25g) tomato purée
1 tbsp (15ml) chopped parsley
½ pt (275ml) natural low-fat yogurt

1. Cook the carrots, onion and garlic in a covered non-stick pan over a low heat for about 10 minutes without browning.

2. Stir in the tomatoes and stock. Season well with the salt and pepper, nutmeg and tomatoe purée. Cover and cook for 30 minutes.

3. Liquidize the soup and store.

4. Just before serving, return to the pan, heat through and stir in the yogurt and parsley. (Alternatively, you might like to pour the soup into a bowl, then top with a swirl of yogurt and parsley.)

Serves: 6   *Calories per serving*: 75

TOMATO AND COURGETTE SOUP

2 tsp (10ml) oil
1 large onion, chopped
1 clove garlic, crushed
14oz (400g) can tomatoes
1lb (450g) courgettes, trimmed and sliced
¼ pt (150ml) water
2 level tbsp (30ml) tomato purée
1 level tsp (5ml) sugar
a few leaves fresh basil, chopped
1 tbsp (15ml) wine vinegar
ground black pepper
4 level tbsp (60ml) natural low-fat yogurt

1. Heat the oil in a large saucepan and cook the onion and garlic until soft, stirring frequently for about 5 minutes.

2. Add the tomatoes, courgettes, water, tomato purée, sugar, basil, vinegar and black pepper. Simmer for 20 minutes or until all the vegetables are tender.

3. Purée in a blender and serve with a swirl of yogurt on top of each portion.

Serves: 4   *Calories per serving*: 90

MARINADE

LEMON MARINADE

1 tbsp (15ml) oil
1 clove garlic, crushed
juice of ½ lemon
ground black pepper
2 tbsp (30ml) chopped fresh herbs (e.g. basil, thyme, parsley, coriander) or ½ level tbsp (7.5ml) mixed dried herbs

Mix all ingredients and spread over meat or fish. Leave to marinate for at least 30 minutes. Cook under the grill.

Serves: 2   *Calories per serving*: 60

VEGETABLES

COURGETTES WITH LIME AND CUMIN

6 small courgettes
4 fl oz (100ml) chicken stock
pinch of ground cumin
salt and freshly ground pepper to taste
juice of 1 lime or small lemon

1. Wash and trim courgettes, cut in half and then into strips about 2in long and ½ in wide.

2. Pour stock into a heavy, non-stick frying pan and bring to the boil.

3. Pile in the courgettes. Grind in black pepper and sprinkle in the cumin. Toss with a wooden spatula until the vegetables are cooked and the stock reduced to almost nothing.

4. Squeeze over the lime or lemon juice, season to taste and serve piping hot.

Serves: 2   *Calories per serving*: 50

(*Note*: You can also cook cauliflower, leeks or green beans this way.)

KEEP YOUR RECORDS HERE

Our volunteers were weighed and measured nine times during the programme. Make a note of your own progress on these pages. Note, too, the change (hopefully for the better!) in your skin, hair and general feeling of well-being.

EXAMPLES

DAY 1   Weight *10* st *10* lb

Measurements: Bust *39in* Waist *29in* Hips *40in*

Skin *Dry, greyish with open pores around nose*

Hair *Dull, split ends, uneven cut, droopy perm*

Well-being *Feel fine until about 4pm,*

      then get tired very easily.

      Generally a bit "off"

DAY 30   Weight *10* st _____ lb

Measurements: Bust *35in* Waist *25in* Hips *38in*

Skin *Glowing, fewer open pores*

Hair *Glossy, a lovely new cut and style*

Well-being *So full of energy that I'm wearing my*

      family out! Every day seems too short.

      I feel great!

DAY 1   Weight _____ st _____ lb

Measurements: Bust _____ Waist _____ Hips _____

Skin _____

Hair _____

Well-being _____

_____

_____

DAY 4   Weight _____ st _____ lb

Measurements: Bust _____ Waist _____ Hips _____

Skin _____

Hair _____

Well-being _____

_____

_____

DAY 7   Weight _____ st _____ lb

Measurements: Bust _____ Waist _____ Hips _____

Skin _____

Hair _____

Well-being _____

_____

_____

DAY 11   Weight _____ st _____ lb

Measurements: Bust _____ Waist _____ Hips _____

Skin _____

Hair _____

Well-being _____

_____

_____

DAY 14   Weight _____ st _____ lb

Measurements: Bust _____ Waist _____ Hips _____

Skin _____

Hair _____

Well-being _____

_____

_____

DAY 18   Weight _____ st _____ lb

Measurements: Bust _____ Waist _____ Hips _____

Skin _____

Hair _____

Well-being _____

_____

_____

DAY 21   Weight _____ st _____ lb

Measurements: Bust _____ Waist _____ Hips _____

Skin _____

Hair _____

Well-being _____

_____

_____

DAY 26   Weight _____ st _____ lb

Measurements: Bust _____ Waist _____ Hips _____

Skin _____

Hair _____

Well-being _____

_____

_____

DAY 30   Weight _____ st _____ lb

Measurements: Bust _____ Waist _____ Hips _____

Skin _____

Hair _____

Well-being _____

_____

_____